Medicine and Society in Late Imperial China

ASIAN
THOUGHT
AND
CULTURE

Sandra A. Wawrytko
General Editor

Vol. 61

PETER LANG
New York • Washington, D.C./Baltimore • Bern
Frankfurt am Main • Berlin • Brussels • Vienna • Oxford

Yüan-ling Chao

Medicine and Society in Late Imperial China

A Study of Physicians in Suzhou, 1600–1850

PETER LANG
New York • Washington, D.C./Baltimore • Bern
Frankfurt am Main • Berlin • Brussels • Vienna • Oxford

Library of Congress Cataloging-in-Publication Data

Chao, Yüan-ling.
Medicine and society in late imperial China: a study
of physicians in Suzhou, 1600–1850 / Yüan-ling Chao.
p. cm. — (Asian thought and culture; v. 61)
Includes bibliographical references and index.
1. Medicine, Chinese—China—Suzhou Shi (Jiangsu Sheng)—History.
2. Confucianism. I. Title. II. Series: Asian thought and culture; v. 61.
[DNLM: 1. History, Modern 1601– —China. 2. Confucianism—history—
China. 3. Physician's Role—history—China. 4. Sociology,
Medical—China. WZ 70 JC6 C5325m 2009]
R603.S89C46 610.951—dc22 2009011342
ISBN 978-1-4331-0381-0
ISSN 0893-6870

Bibliographic information published by **Die Deutsche Bibliothek**.
Die Deutsche Bibliothek lists this publication in the "Deutsche
Nationalbibliografie"; detailed bibliographic data is available
on the Internet at http://dnb.ddb.de/.

The paper in this book meets the guidelines for permanence and durability
of the Committee on Production Guidelines for Book Longevity
of the Council of Library Resources.

29 Broadway, 18th floor, New York, NY 10006
www.peterlang.com

Printed in Germany

To the memory of my father

Chao Chüan-ying
趙傳纓

scholar and gentleman

TABLE OF CONTENTS

Part II: Medicine in Late Imperial Suzhou

ACKNOWLEDGMENTS

MANY people provided invaluable advice and support in the long process of turning this work into a book. First and foremost, I would like to acknowledge my gratitude to Benjamin Elman and Francesca Bray for their support and encouragement over the course of this project, and throughout my career. Richard von Glahn has always been supportive and a source of inspiration. I am much in debt to Nathan Sivin for his continued interest in my work and his generosity in the time and guidance he is willing to give to young scholars. He graciously read over my original dissertation and offered incisive comments and suggestions. Carol Benedict also read over my entire dissertation with care and provided valuable advice on revisions. I am appreciative of Kathryn Bernhardt, Philip Huang, Herman Ooms, James Tong and Robert Frank for their guidance and support. Chang Chia-feng and Chu Ping-yi were generous in sharing their work and commenting on segments of the manuscript. The comments and constructive criticism from an anonymous reviewer has been very helpful in rethinking some of the issues. My colleagues in the History Department at Middle Tennessee State University have helped with my English, as well as provide moral support. I am deeply grateful to Martha Harroun Foster, Mary Hoffschwelle, and Susan Myers-Shirk. All remaining mistakes, of course, are mine.

It gives me great pleasure to acknowledge the assistance and hospitality that I received over time at the various libraries in different countries. The initial research for my dissertation was generously supported by a Dissertation Research Fellowship in Chinese Studies by the Joint Committee on Chinese Studies of the American Council of Learned Societies and the Social Science Research Council (ACLS/SSRC). This research grant that allowed me to spend one year at Kyoto University's Jimbun Kagaku Kenkyûjo, and travel to Tokyo and Taiwan for research. Subsequent writing was supported by a UCLA Center for Chinese Studies Dissertation Fellowship.

The staff at various libraries have always cheerfully assisted me in my requests and provided help in finding materials. These libraries include Kyoto University's Jimbum kagaku kenkûjo, Tokyo University's Tôyô Bunko, the Fu Ssu-nian library at the Academia Sinica in Taiwan, the library at the China Academy of Traditional Chinese Medicine (Zhongguo zhongyi yanjiu yuan) in Beijing, the East Asian Library and the Gest Collection at Princeton University, and the Richard C. Rudolph East Asian Library at UCLA. During my stay in Kyoto, Ono Katsuko, served not only as mentor, but also provided warm hospitality and guidance.Yamada Keiji of the International Research Institute on Japanese Culture was extremely kind to me and unceasingly encouraging in my work. I was also privileged to sit in the Ming-Qing Society and Culture seminar at the Jimbun, and Sakade Yoshinobu's *neidan* seminar. I also benefited from discussions with Fuma Susumu of Kyoto University, whose work on charitable organizations helped me better understand local gentry and society in late imperial times. At the Academia Sinica in Taiwan I enjoyed the hospitality of Angela Leung Ki-Chi and Liu Ts'ui-jung. Martin Heijdra of Princeton University's East Asian Library and the Gest Collection has provided much support and research assistance during my visits. My stay at the library at the China Academy of Traditional Chinese Medicine (Zhongguo zhongyi yanjiu yuan) was greatly facilitated by Zhu Jianping, Vice-Director of the China Institute for the History of Medicine and Medical Literature. The Librarian Qiu Jian also gave me much needed access to the rare books collection.

My summer trip to Beijing in 2002 was generously support by a Faculty Research and Creative Projects award from MTSU. I wish to recognize the support from John McDaniel, Dean of the College of Liberal Arts at MTSU for my book project, and to the Graduate School at MTSU for generously funding the subvention costs of the book.

Grateful acknowledgement is hereby made to the editor, Hans Ulrich Vogel, of *East Asian Science, Technology, and Medicine*, for permission to use parts of my article "The Ideal Physician in Late Imperial China: The Question of *Sanshi*."

Finally, to Yu Chia-yun, Yu Chiu-tien, and Chao Yüan-tsien, my deepest appreciation for their tolerance and patience as I labored through this project. Special thanks to Chia-yun for not only being my valuable proof reader, but uncomplainingly looked after my growing menagerie of pets while I was gone. And, to my loyal cat Mimi, who, while battling cancer and chronic kidney disease, rarely fails to keep me company at nights when I work, warming my lap and heart.

ABBREVIATIONS

CZWXZ	*Chongzhen Wuxian zhi* 崇禎吳縣志
CZXZ	*Changzhou xianzhi* 長洲縣志
DMHD	*Da Ming hui dian* 大明會典
DQHD	*Da Qing hui dian* 大清會典
GJTSJC	*Gujin tushu jichen* 古今圖書集成
GSZ	*Gusu zhi* 姑蘇志
HMJSWB	*Huang ming jing shi wen bian* 皇明經世文編
JSLDYRZ	Chen Daojin and Xue Weitao, *Jiangsu lidai yirenzhi* 江蘇歷代醫人志
MGWXZ	*Mingguo Wuxian zhi.* 民國吳縣志
MHY	*Ming hui yao* 明會要
MS	*Mingshii* 明史
MSL	*Ming shi lu* 明實錄 (Veritable Records of the Ming Emperors): *Ming taizu shilu* 明太祖實錄 (MTZSL); *Ming shizong shilu* 明世宗實錄 (MSZSL); *Ming muzong shilu* 明穆宗實錄(MMZSL)
QCTD	*Qingchao tongdian* 清朝通典
QJL	*Qingjialu* 清嘉錄
QSG	*Qingshi gao* 清史稿

SZFZ	*Suzhou fu zhi* 蘇州府志
WMBY	*Wumen biaoyin* 吳門表隱
YDZ	*Yuan dian zhang* 元典章
YS	*Yuan shi* 元史

INTRODUCTION

Toward a History of Medicine in Late Imperial China

WALK into a Chinese pharmacy today and one will find, in addition to hundreds of drawers of ingredients for herbal decoctions, packaged medicines for everyday ills. Often these packaged medicines will tout their efficacy based on *laofang* (traditional formula), or attribute their reliability and value to a historically famous physician. Therefore it is not unusual to find images of Qing dynasty (1644–1911) Suzhou physician Ye Tianshi (ca.1690–1760), or the seventeenth century pharmacologist Li Shizhen (1518–1593) on boxes of medicine. However, walk into a pharmacy in the West, and one will not find images of Edward Jenner or William Harvey on bottles of aspirin. Rather, the latest medical research and findings are the basis for the value and efficacy of the medicines sold. Similarly, in the training of physicians, a survey of modern textbooks used in teaching in traditional Chinese medical academies invariably finds discussions of canonical works such as the *Huangdi neijing* (Inner Canon of the Yellow Emperor), the *Shennong bencaojing* (*Materia Medica* of the Divine Husbandman, compiled around late first or second century A.D.), and various "schools" of medicine that developed over the centuries. On the other hand, one will not find a study of the *Hippocratic Corpus* a requirement within the curriculum of Western medical schools. This underscores the different ways of legitimation between Western and Chinese classical medical traditions.

This book examines the issue of legitimation in medicine within the fluid and multi-layered classical medical landscape of late imperial China. I weave together cultural factors, economic trends, and state strategies with developments in medical theories that were informed by practice and regional specificities. This shows a vibrant medical landscape in late imperial China and reveals that medical ideas and practices resist simple classification and drawing of definitive boundaries. It also shows that was much fluidity between state strategies, elite discourse, formation of an orthodoxy based on text and lineage, medical theories and popular ideas and practices concerning illness and healing.

The formation of lineages and orthodoxy in classical medicine, and state strategies of patronizing popular physicians and healing legends did not, however, create a homogeneous medical culture. Instead, I argue that imperial patronage of physicians and sponsorship of an orthodox lineage in classical medicine, and the *ruyi*'s (Confucian physicians) efforts in forging a professional identity failed to dictate ideas and practices of medicine. In a study of the god Wutong, Richard von Glahn shows that while there was exchange of ideas between elite and peasant classes, the elite did not monopolize the dialogue as the lower classes produced their own narrative.[1] Prasenjit Duara, in his study of Guangdi, shows how different social groups, ranging from the village at the bottom to the imperial state at the top, impose their own meanings on cultural symbols and figures. He refers to this layering of meaning over time as "superscription."[2] This allows different groups to ascribe their own meanings to symbols. Thus we will see in medicine, symbols such as the *sanhuang* (Three Emperors) and their temple were ascribed special meanings by different groups. What emerged was layers of narrative and different channels of legitimation.

The rise and increasing influence of the *wenbing* (warm factor) school had much to do with the cultural dominance and economic affluence of the lower Yangzi area in the Ming and Qing dynasties. Physicians of this school claimed legitimacy not only through the authority of the textual tradition, but also by asserting theoretical and therapeutic separation from the *shanghan* school based on observation and specificities of the southern locality.

In this book, I use the term classical medical tradition instead of traditional Chinese medicine in order to avoid confusion with what is referred to as Traditional Chinese Medicine (TCM) in the West. TCM was introduced into the West as an organized system of medicine compatible with modern science and technology by the Chinese government in the 1950s. Recent works by Bridie Andrews, Elisabeth Hsu, and Kim Taylor have all examined the construction of TCM in China.[3] Mao proclaimed traditional Chinese medicine to be one of the great treasures of China, but he also wanted to package it as scientific to both within and without China. But, as reflected in the modern consumer economy, tradition still figures prominently even in TCM.

Medicine in Late Imperial Jiangnan

The vitality of the medical landscape in late imperial Jiangnan[4] owes much to its economic and cultural developments. Recent scholarship has illuminated the economic transformations in the region, including the influx of silver and the monetarization of the economy.[5] The link to global trade encouraged cash crops and commercialization of handicraft industries such as silk and tea. Dynastic transition and epidemics contributed to a half century of population decline and depressed economy,[6] but recovery was evident by the end of the seventeenth century. Jiangnan in particular enjoyed a robust recovery and economic growth.[7] This economic prosperity in the Jiangnan region also led to population increase and rise in living standards. Kenneth Pomeranz speculated that the average adult male's grain consumption in the Jiangnan region during the eighteenth century was around 3,181 calories per day.[8]

This economic affluence led to thriving urban centers and contributed to extensive and profound social and cultural changes. These included a more fluid class structure, the growth of a vibrant urban culture, booming publishing networks, and a different conception of wealth. How all these developments helped to shape the medical landscape and provide the context for the discourse over legitimation will be a central theme in the book.

One significant development in medicine, as reflected in contemporary records, was the rise in the number of practicing physicians. This was due not only to increased population in the region but also to two other factors. The first was the intensified competition in the civil service examinations that was closely tied to the economic and cultural rise of Jiangnan. Benjamin has shown in his studies that Jiangsu and Zhejiang produced the highest numbers of *jinshi* (presented candidates).[9] However, quotas for the examinations also meant that it became increasingly difficult to pass the civil service examinations. Thus, it was not uncommon to find in the biographies of physicians that most had started out as aspiring examination candidates. Only after repeated failures did many abandon their quests and take up medicine. Second, the number of clientele also increased as affluent merchants and gentry could afford the classically trained physicians. Subsequently, as the field of practicing physicians became more crowded, the contestation for the claim as the best qualified became more intense. leading to lively efforts to negotiate qualifications of the ideal physician through literary debates explored in Chapter One. These included debates over the proper interpretation of *sanshi* (three generations) in the ancient classic *Liji* (Book of Rites), and the correct identity of the figures in the *sidajia* (Four Major Schools). A booming publishing network and lively literary scene facilitated these efforts. The correspondences and writings of physicians show that they traveled in the region, sometimes to treat patients, and sometimes to visit other physicians. The vast trade and market networks undoubtedly facilitated and encouraged these travels and exchanges.

The focus on socioeconomic and cultural developments in shaping the medical landscape does not mean that the state would be neglected. On the contrary, I contend that the state played an important function in the process of legitimation in two ways. First, it patronized the canonical tradition that traced its lineage back to the in two ways. First, it patronized the canonical tradition that traced its lineage back to the Yellow Emperor through compilation of medical collections as well as in the ritual worship of the Three Emperors (Huangdi, Shennong, and Fuxi). Second, the Qing dynasty's support of the evidential research movement helped to facilitate research into the medical classics and livened discussions over proper diagnosis and therapy. This played an important role in shaping the *wenbing* (warm factor) versus *shanghan* (cold damage) debate. Overall, elevation of the canonical tradition lent credence to the idea of the Confucian physician as the ideal fit into their strategies of legitimation.

In the second part of the book I narrow my focus to the city of Suzhou, i.e., the counties of Wu, Changzhou, and Yuanhe,[10] not only because of the impressive assembly of physicians in the area, but also it was the locus of activities of the physicians central to the development of the *wenbing* (warm factor) theory in medicine. It provides for a unique opportunity to explore the interrelationship between medicine and the economic and cultural developments of the region, the networks of physicians and literati, and the layered relationship between state and local practice.

The increasing participation of elites in medical practice in late imperial China contributed to efforts toward demarcating boundaries of inclusion and exclusion. This was accomplished by defining the qualities of an ideal physician—that of a *ruyi* (Confucian physician). The ideal emphasized an ethical model, intellectual intelligence shaped by training in the classics, and membership based upon specialized knowledge that came from the classical tradition. This process fostered the development of a group consciousness, facilitated by the social and literary networks among the elite. I argue therefore that the physicians in late imperial Jiangnan were creating a professional identity for themselves, not through institutional or legal means, but through cultural and social strategies.[11]

Although much of the discussion focuses on the elite physicians, the formation of a medical orthodoxy, and contestation among different groups of physicians, the heterogeneous nature and layered practices of medicine meant that the elite physicians never were able to monopolize the dialogue and impose a uniform authority over notions of health and healing practices. There was undoubtedly a wider dissemination of medical knowledge and the popularity of medical books fostered acceptance of classical theories. In her study on the women of the Zhang family, Susan Mann observes that, "All this publishing activity points not just to the spread of medical knowledge among the elite but also to the dissemination of that knowledge among literate commoners."[12] However, as will be discussed in the following section, classical medicine had absorbed and assimilated diverse traditions over the centuries, and the Confucian cloak that late imperial physicians attempted to use for representation of an orthodoxy actually masked a tradition that was eclectic from the beginning.

Classical Chinese Medicine in Late Imperial China: Schools, Lineages, and Orthodoxy

The heterogeneous nature of Chinese medicine is shaped by the roots of its formation, where folk religious rituals, diverse local notions of health and healing, and accumulation of practical experiences all played a role. Donald Harper found that the earliest medical texts that were recovered from the Mawangdui tombs "provide evidence of an earlier stage in the formation of the physiological and pathological theories that support acupuncture therapy in the *Huangdi neijing*."[13] Many of the texts were concerned with *yangsheng* (nourishing life) techniques that were later adopted by Daoism. Thus what is often regarded as Daoist perceptions of the body often preceded the appearance of Daoism. Vivienne Lo has shown that *yangsheng* texts helped to shape the canonical tradition that was to emerge later in the Western Han (202 B.C.–9 A.D.).[14]

Sivin has commented that in China since the early times, there has been a tendency for "identification with a group and aspiration toward an imagined orthodoxy."[15] The compilation of the *Huangdi neijing* reflected its incorporation of the notions of *yin/yang* and five phases into the interpretative framework. These were basic principles of dualism and systematic correspondence to various aspects of nature that showed a belief in the ability of humans to understand nature based on a system of natural laws. Influence of the four seasons was also heavily emphasized in the text.[16] The formation of schools (*jia*) in early medicine emerged as the transmission of knowledge came to be revolved around written texts, and the passing down of the knowledge is connected to receiving these texts by disciples from teachers, often ritually sanctioned. This tradition of the formation of schools around revered texts of legendary figures can be found in Confucian schools as well as those in fields such as mathematics. In medicine there were at least three identifiable schools related to the Yellow Emperor, Bian Que, and Master Bai. The classical medical canon in medicine that is attributed to the legendary sage Huangdi (Yellow Emperor) was an eclectic collection of writings that reflected different traditions and accounts for some of the contradictions that seem to permeate the text. The *Huangdi neijing* (Inner Canon of the Yellow Emperor) became the sacred text of an orthodox tradition that evolved over time, reflecting a triumph of the *Huangdi* school. The various schools that developed over the centuries may differ over causation and therapy for diseases, they all, however, look to the *Huangdi neijing* as the source of their correctness. Subsequent medical texts such as *Nanjing* and Huangfu Mi's *Zhenjiu jiayijing* provides elaboration on practical applications of healing techniques.

A major period of development in the formation of an orthodoxy came in the Song, Jin and Yuan periods. This was facilitated greatly by the personal interests of the Northern Song emperors as well as an urgent need to respond to the outbreak of epidemics from the eleventh to the twelfth centuries. Asaf Goldschmidt has effectively shown how these developments contributed to increasing state patronage of medicine, both in printing of books and setting up of institutions.[17] This period not only witnessed the emergence of various schools of thought and practice, but the patronage of the Song government in the compilation and editing of texts served to elevate the *Huangdi neijing* to a canonical status. The subsequent formation of the *sanhuang* (Three Emperors) lineage and the Yuan government's formal ritual worship of the *sanhuang* as the progenitors of the medical tradition solidified the orthodox status of the *Huangdi* school and merged the textual tradition with the ritual tradition of worship.

Another text that came into prominence was the *Shanghanlun* by the Later Han physician Zhang Zhongjing. The text however remained rather obscure until the Song dynasty when printing by the government led to

increasing interest. Editing and commentaries on the text led to the emergence of the *shanghan* school that focused on therapy inspired by the author's experiences with epidemic diseases. The formation of the *shanghan* school thus did not gain momentum until then and became well-established in the Ming and Qing.

Zhang Zhongjing's *Shanghanlun* provided the theoretical and therapeutic stimulation for the development of the *wenbing* school. The latter traced its theoretical origins to the *Huangdi neijing*, but it was the effort to establish a separate theory of diagnosis and therapy for heat factor and epidemic diseases from the *shanghan* school that distinguished it in late imperial Jiangnan. This process was shaped by the participation in medicine by increasing numbers of Confucian physicians as well as by practical experience of practitioners in their treatment of patients. The regional specificities and experience with epidemics helped to foster new ways of thinking and practice among the *wenbing* physicians. The birth and maturation of the *wenbing* school involved first a claim to legitimacy by tracing its origins to the *Huangdi neijing*, then secondly, because it had been placed under the *shanghan* category, formulation of an independent theory on diagnosis and therapy. Wu Youxing and his theory of *liqi* invading the body through the mouth and nose played a key role in forging a break with the *shanghan* tradition, which emphasized the importance of seasonal changes in causing illnesses. This process in the growth of the *wenbing* school also involved scholarly discourse over the authenticity of the work *Shanghanlun*. However, as Marta Hanson has shown, the rise of the *wenbing* also was closely tied to the increasing dominance of the south, built upon a notion of fundamental differences between northern and southern bodies.[18]

Medical orthodoxy however was not merely based on texts. We can also discern a ritual orthodoxy in the worshipping of the Three Emperors as well as famous physicians in the *sanhuang miao* (Temple of the Three Emperors) beginning in the Yuan dynasty. Many of the famous physicians included in the *sanhuang miao* were already worshipped by people at the local levels, but their incorporation into the temple created a state sponsored worshipping of the practitioners of medicine. It was an attempt on part of the state to extend authority and influence in the practice of medicine, and at the same time an acknowledgement of the importance of practice in medicine. The growing numbers of Confucian physicians in late imperial times contributed to an increased interest in the elevation and protection of the orthodoxy traced to the Three Emperors.

The complex competition among the different schools that emerged after the Song, Jin, and Yuan periods also contributed to an effort in the elevation of Zhang Zhongjing, author of the *Shanghanlun*, as *yisheng* (medical sage) in the Ming and Qing. Originally one of four schools, he was elevated to the head of a lineage of medicine to match the veneration of Confucius in the Confucian schools of thought. However, the veneration of Zhang Zhongjing was not embraced by others. His "rival" among the commoners was Sun Simiao (581-682), a Tang dynasty (618-906) physician who was elevated as the Medicine King.

We find not only a textual orthodoxy but also a ritual orthodoxy patronized by the state. However, as my research will show, the ritual worship of medical practitioners were dictated not by the state, but by popular sentiment. In the case of the *sanhuang miao,* they were not as popular as the *yaowang miao* and some were converted into the latter. Although Sun Simiao was often regarded as the *yaowang*, there was no set criteria and standard. Here, we see popular beliefs and traditions ascribing meaning to images and spaces that the elite attempted to define. The state's effort in establishing an orthodox ritual tradition in medicine was maintained within a narrow range and did not extend beyond the elite level. The fact that it was Zhang Zhongjing and not the legendary Yellow Emperor that was characterized as the medical sage reflected the importance of practice. Medicine was not only an intellectual exercise, but also a technical skill.

Medicine East and West: The Issue of Professionalization

> "The human body contains blood, phlegm, yellow bile and black bile. These are the things that make up its constitution and cause its pains and health. Health is primarily that state in which these constituent substances are in the correct proportion to each other, both in strength and quantity, and are well mixed. Pain occurs when one of the substances presents either a deficiency or an excess, or is separated in the body and not mixed with the others."
>
> The Nature of Man" in the *Hippocratic Corpus*[19]

> "Thus mankind should correspond to this system: the Yin and Yang of man are (arranged in the order) that on the outside there is Yang, and inside there is Yin. Yin and Yang of the human body (are arranged) that Yang is in back and Yin is within the front part. Yin and Yang of the (five) viscera and the (six) bowels are (arranged) that the viscera are Yin and the hollow organs are Yang. All of the five viscera, liver, heart, spleen, lungs and kidneys, are Yin; and all of the five hollow organs, gall-bladder, stomach, lower intestines, bladder, and the three burning spaces, are all Yang.

> The reason why we must know (the rule of) the Yin within the Yin and (the rule of) the Yang within the Yang is that the diseases of Winter are located in (the region of)Yang and the diseases of Summer in (the region of)Yin; the diseases of Spring are located in (the region of) Yin and the diseases of Fall in (the region of) Yang."
>
> "Treatise on the Truth of the Golden Box" in *Huangdi neijing suwen,* Ch.4[20]

The human body is seen and experienced through social and cultural lenses. Since mankind cannot escape from afflictions of diseases of the body, medicine is shaped by two activities universal to humankind: as a technical skill to cure illnesses, and as an intellectual activity to develop a coherent theory with which to explain body, health, and illness. These interconnected activities are, however, rooted in the culture from which they emerge, and therefore, medical systems can only be understood within the particular social, cultural, economic, and political context from which they evolve.[21] As Charles Rosenberg pointed out, the phrase "social history of medicine" is redundant and tautological, since all medicine is essentially social.[22] Thus in view of the fact that medicine is rooted in the society in which it emerged, can there be common concepts that can be applied to different cultures? What would such an exercise contribute? In the study of the relationship between physicians and society, one of the key concepts that emerged in the field of the history of medicine is the idea of "professionalization." Can this be used in the Chinese context? What useful function can it serve? I believe that it can contribute to a better understanding of different cultural traditions if we do not try to apply it as a broad universal concept, but rather a key processes in which institutional regulation, networking, and exclusivity that enabled the physicians to claim a professional identity. By examining processes, we can have a better understanding of the ways of legitimation in China where the literati physicians strove to create an exclusive identity and privileges for themselves.

When we examine the process of professionalization in the West, it is clear that it was rooted in very different social, political, and cultural spheres. The history of medicine as a branch of historical inquiry is very much related to the rise of the medical profession and its increasing dominance within the structure of power. The medical system as known in Western societies today, has come into existence only fairly recently, and it was not so long ago that hospitals were considered as places of filth and death, and surgeons earned little more respect or money than barbers. This transition reflected the gradual professionalization of medicine in Europe beginning in the seventeenth and eighteenth centuries and an increasing dominance of the medical profession within the structure of power. Freidson has commented that "medicine has displaced the law and the ministry from their once dominant positions."[23] Developing the study of the history of medicine as a legitimate historical inquiry further legitimizes and enhances the prestige of the profession itself. Therefore it is not surprising that the initial phase of the study of the history of medicine, largely undertaken by physicians, was the study of the victorious march of scientific medicine over previously unbeatable illnesses and diseases. It was mainly a chronicle of the great men in medicine and their achievements.

One of the more important works in this changing perspective is by Michel Foucault. In *The Birth of the Clinic*, a study on the advent of modern scientific medicine, Foucault declared the emergence of what he termed the new medical 'gaze' in nineteenth century Europe by looking back into the traditional medicine of the seventeenth and eighteenth centuries. Nosological considerations were the main concerns in traditional medicine rather than the examination of the patients themselves. The sociopolitical climate of the French Revolution harbored the seeds of the development of the anatomo-clinical style that emerged from about 1790–1830, where patients were treated in hospitals for specific pathological symptoms. The growth of urban population during this period increased the need for hygiene and thus entailed certain authoritarian medical interventions and controls, particularly at prisons, ships, hospitals and so on. Therefore medicine assumed "an increasingly important place in the administrative system and the machinery of power, a role which is constantly widened and strengthened throughout the eighteenth century."[24]

This transition, Foucault finds, is also related to the change in the conception of death and disease. He comments, "Disease breaks away from the metaphysic of evil, to which it had been related for centuries, and it finds in the visibility of death the full form in which its content appears in positive terms."[25] He went on to explain "[I]t is when death became the concrete a priori of medical experience that death could detach itself from counter-nature and become embodied in the living bodies of individuals."[26] The change in status and power of the medical profession is also well documented in the literature on Western history of medicine.[27]

It is well accepted that medical professionalization plays a central role in societies today. There have been numerous studies on the professionalization of practitioners of medicine in America and Europe.[28] Given a different set of status relationships and structure of power between medicine and society in late imperial China, the question arises as to whether physicians in China at the time could be considered a professional group.[29]The professionaliza-

tion of the physicians in the West has been closely related to its emergence in the structure of power both politically and socially. Although this was not the case in China, where the physicians never attained a dominant position in the political and social structure, I would nevertheless argue that there were factors that constituted a process of professionalization of medicine in late imperial China..

For some scholars, professionalization is generally understood as the presence of a systematic body of knowledge, authority derived from monopolization of specialized knowledge, and recognition by society in the form of privileges and power, code of ethics, and a sense of community. Here I propose to look at the formation of a professional community among the physicians through their attempts to create boundaries of inclusion and exclusion. The influx of the elite into the group of physicians in late imperial China hastened this process by developing a group consciousness, facilitated by the social and literary networks among the elite, emphasis on an ethical model, and membership based upon specialized knowledge.

Regarding late imperial Chinese society, the study by Benjamin Elman on Jiangnan's academic community shows that, even though the transformation toward more formal scholarly occupations and roles was not yet complete during the Qing, the group of scholars involved in evidential research (*kaozheng*) scholarship[30] were undergoing a process of professionalization.[31] Dardess in his study of Confucianism in the Ming dynasty also discusses the formation of professional elites and sees the use of Confucianism as a form of professional knowledge.[32] However in his effort to portray the Confucians as a national professional elite to explain the autocracy of the Ming state, Dardess has ignored the diversity within the group of Confucians and the changes that were underway intellectually and socially in Ming society.

The question of the professionalization of medicine has been a major theme in the comparison of medicine in the East and West, as evidenced by the volume produced by the International Symposium on the Comparative History of Medicine—East and West.[33] Paul Unschuld, in his chapter examining the study of medicine in China and the question of professionalization, uses the resource model and defines it as "a process during which the control of a given group of health-care providers over resources pertaining to health care is increased."[34]

The classical medical tradition in China is closely related to the dominant Confucian tradition. There have been different opinions concerning the merits of the close alliance between medicine, especially classical medicine, with Confucian intellectual traditions and institutions. Ralph Croizier commented that Chinese medicine was "perhaps too well integrated into its larger culture, for the same factors that inhibited scientific development in the culture as a whole acted to retard the further development of medicine."[35] Manfred Porkert claims that "from the Sung period, the Great Medical Office became a permanent institution, receiving some 300 medical students; and the academy-trained physicians inherited some of the prestige, but not the social independence, of the [earlier] Taoist practitioners. To the transmission and continuous evolution of Chinese medical science, its institutionalization and integration into the Confucian administration was a doubtful benefit...The qualitative decline of Chinese medical science, and with it the social downgrading of its practitioners, began under the Yuan in the fourteenth century. It continued under the Ming and became rife by the middle of the Ch'ing era..."[36] Thus both Croizier and Porkert believe that close association with the Confucian tradition had a negative effect upon medical development in China. They were both, in a way, still caught in the web of Joseph Needham's 'why not' question.

On the other hand, Joseph Needham, although often still approaching Chinese science from the "why not" perspective, had a different opinion on the influence of Confucian culture upon medical developments. He believed that "the whole history of the social position of doctors might be summarized as the passage from the *wu*, a sort of technological servitor, to the *shih*, a particular kind of scholar, clad in the full dignity of the Confucian intellectual...There was a general move throughout the Middle Ages to raise the intellectual standing of the physician...The gradual change was important, for it ensured the existence of considerable numbers of physicians well educated in general literature and with greater culture than their predecessors had possessed."[37]

Where does the physician fit into the picture? Are they part of the "great tradition" or do they belong to the "little tradition"? The answer is that the division itself is arbitrary and analytically flawed. As mentioned above, the *yi* can be divided roughly into the elite and folk tradition, or literate and non-literate. However, although it was classically educated Confucian physicians who were held in high esteem, there was considerable interaction with other medical practitioners and the line between the two was quite fluid.

Like the Greek physician, traditionally the Chinese physician was considered an artisan. Bian Que was said to have traveled from place to place and either became a pediatrician, geriatrician, or gynecologist according to the needs of his surroundings. This feature, that of an itinerant physician, was to remain until the late imperial period. In the dynastic histories, biographies of the physicians could be found under the *fangji* (craft) and *yishu* (arts) categories. Similarly, in the local gazetteers, they were often classified under *yishu*. Thus physicians were included, listed with astronomers, geomancers, artists, and other types of craftsmen.

The gap that existed between the literate and the non-literate physicians was wide, and the Confucian physician probably had more in common with a fellow Confucian than with the itinerant physician who wandered from place to place. However, to define a horizontal classification of physicians obscures the vertical connections and the roots of medical knowledge and practice in traditional China. There is however also a problem with the term "Confucian." First it conveyed a false sense of unity among a particular group of physicians, and, secondly, it linked them closely to an intellectual tradition that itself is diverse and undergoing change. What I show in my study is that the "Confucianization" of medicine by elite physicians must be examined alongside of the ways in which medicine was actually practiced to understand the dynamics of change and transformation in the medical landscape.

In the formal structure of social and political institutions, there is little doubt that the physicians did not occupy a position at the high levels. The formal Confucian hierarchy relegated the physician to the position of the artisan. Putting on the cloak of the Confucian scholar thus elevated the physician within the Confucian hierarchy. However when we look closely into physicians and their position in society, the picture becomes less clear. The fluidity of society in the Ming and Qing periods, especially in the Jiangnan area, also brought about different attitudes towards class and society, and, during the late imperial period, popular conceptions of the physician underwent changes. This book is an attempt to look at the physician not just from the point of view of the Confucian scholar, but also from the medical tradition itself and including how popular perceptions of the physician changed.

The transmission of medical knowledge will be discussed in detail in Chapter 3, here I would like to point out that in traditional China, medical knowledge was transmitted through both the oral and the literate tradition. The early Bian Que received the transmission of medical knowledge from Chang Sang Jun. The process involved not only the confirmation of the worthiness of Bian Que to receive the knowledge, but also shamanistic and religious ceremonies. The process of medical training for the physician Chunyu Yi involved three stages: oral transmission, confirmation of his ability, and study of ancient texts and practice.[38] Medical knowledge was often transmitted from father to son or through apprenticeship. There were indications that observation and practical experience were important in the training of a physician in addition to the study of texts. The famous Suzhou physician Ye Tianshi was said to have sought the guidance of thirteen teachers after the death of his father.

The Confucian physicians often emphasized textual transmission, while the hereditary physicians such as Ye Tianshi placed more emphasis upon practical experience and personal transmissions. This led to tensions between the two groups and found expression in debates over the interpretation of the ancient classic *Liji* (Book of Rites) where the *Quli* declared "one does not take the medicine of those without the three generations."(*yibusanshi bufuqiyao*) Confucian physicians believed that the three generations here referred to the three ancient medical classics representing the three medical traditions, emphasizing theory and knowledge, whereas the hereditary physicians believed it to be a reference to three generations of physicians within the family, placing an emphasis on experience.

The tremendous social and economic changes that occurred during the late Ming and Qing periods brought about significant developments in the medical tradition as well. There was a greater fluidity in the society where medicine became an attractive alternative for some families. The Jiangnan region emerged not only as the economic heartland of late imperial China, but economic wealth translated into cultural resources, and Jiangnan became the cultural center that produced the highest number of successful examination candidates. It was also here that we find the largest concentration of physicians. This is not surprising given the increase in population and the need for medical care. Yet it also enabled the emergence of a "community" of physicians who not only practiced medicine, but who also actively engaged in discussions on aspects of the development of medical theories and therapy, contributing to the rise of a new school, the *wenbing* (warm factor) school.

Medicine in the History of Medicine

In the decades since the pioneering studies of Joseph Needham and Lu Gwei-djen, the "High Ancestors" in the history of Chinese science and medicine, the field has moved beyond the "Needham Question"[39] towards a social and cultural history approach that pioneer historian of medicine, Henry Sigerist, called for in the 1940s.[40] Much of this shift can be attributed to a "second generation" of scholars, including Sakade Yoshinobu, Yamada Keiji and Nathan Sivin, who approached Chinese science and medicine by situating them within China's cultural and political milieu.[41]

More recent scholarship has contributed to a more social and cultural approach to medicine. Robert Hyme's study on physician status and strategies from the Song to Yuan has been valuable to my study of Ming–Qing physician and family strategies in career selection.[42] In addition to Asaf Goldschmidt's study of the changes in medicine during the Northern Song, T.J. Hinrichs's work also facilitates our understanding of Song dynasty medical institutions and customs.[43] Charlotte Furth's study places medicine within the intellectual and social context and illuminates how class and gender boundaries are negotiated.[44] Angela Leung's exploration of the state in late imperial medical education and institutions has shed much light on state involvement in medicine in Ming and Qing[45] Yili Wu's study of the Bamboo Grove Monastery's gynecological texts in Qing China illuminated different ways of legitimation and how a practitioner creates identity.[46] Marta Hanson's work on medicine in the lower Yangzi region and the *wenbing* school has been most helpful in examining the rise and development of this important medical school.[47] Joanna Grant's textual study of the physician Wang Ji 's practice in Huizhou brings into focus a deeper understanding the medical practice of a physician.[48]

All these studies have begun to deal with the issue of the place of medicine within the history.[49] The issue for the China field relates to what Sivin referred to as the "Awesome Taboo"[50]—the reluctance (by scholars in humanities) to make use of primary texts and sources in science, technology, and medicine. Benjamin Elman's work on science in China represent the first pioneering effort to bridge the gap between science and the humanities and to forge a discourse between the two fields, for each has much to benefit from a constructive dialogue.[51]

The other side of the problem is what Elman referred to as a "Science Taboo," where scientists, in much of the same way, are unwilling to engage in discussion with historians in the field.[52] This dichotomy in medicine is complicated by the different approaches to the field by those working in China and those trained in the West. While in the West, ethnographic studies such as those of Judith Farquhar and work by historians such as Sivin and Paul Unschuld contributed to a shift toward social and cultural approaches, on mainland China in the study of the history of medicine remained very much in the hands of physicians who were eager to showcase Traditional Chinese Medicine (TCM) as a practice with a long and venerable history, and highlight the scientific effort to merge Chinese and Western medicine (*zhongxi hebi*). Most of those who engaged in the history of medicine in China were trained in traditional medicine and were practitioners of TCM,[53] whereas most of those engaged in this field in the West were mostly trained in history, anthropology, or sociology.[54] Thus even though there have been attempts to bridge the gap between the two, there is not much true dialogue.

Integrating medicine into the history of medicine is important in that it allows for a more nuanced understanding of medicine's place within the larger historical context. It is also important because medicine is, after all, a technical skill. My book aims to begin a small step towards this goal by integrating medicine into a social and cultural analysis.

It is perhaps a less daunting task for the history of medicine in China to include medicine into the discussion as the language used in medicine remained integrated with the intellectual and religious traditions, and practitioners, especially elite physicians, shared with the literati a similar outlook and classical training. Therefore there was not the growing divergence in language in medicine that created a separate scientific elite as in the West.

In my book I hope to bring about a deeper understanding of the relationship between medicine and society in late imperial China through a historical study of the ways of legitimation in medicine in late imperial Jiangnan and a focused study of Suzhou physicians. Much of the information is found in local gazetteers, dynastic histories, various *biji*, private compilations of biographies, as well as medical treatises written by the physicians themselves. The nature of the sources means that we have much more information on the elite physicians than the beliefs and practices of the commoners, but this does not mean that the latter were voiceless. We find the voices of the common people in the meanings they ascribed to spaces such as the Temple of the Three Emperors and powers they endowed upon historical figures.

The book is divided into two parts. Part I provides an analysis of the multi-layered ways of legitimation in medicine within the cultural and economic region of Jiangnan. I show how the networks of publishing and fluidity of movement allowed for intensified interaction among physicians, who used these effectively to foster a professional identity. Their efforts intertwined with the state's attempt in patronage of medicine by the formalization of an orthodoxy in medicine. Woven into this dynamic medical landscape was the growing maturation of a school that claimed legitimacy through the canonical textual tradition, and new theories and practice closely tied to the geography of the south. Chapter one examines the interaction with the intellectual traditions, and the construction of the idea of a Confucian physician; Chapter two looks at medicine's relationship with the state through an in-depth study of the *sanhuang miao* (Temple of the Three

Emperors); and Chapter Three traces the development of medical theories and practices and the rise of the *wenbing* (warm factor school) that was dominant in the region. Part II focuses on the city of Suzhou, providing a micro-study of the themes addressed in Part I. Chapter four analyzes Suzhou physicians and their writings within the broad medical tradition; Chapter five takes a local perspective of medicine's relationship with the state through an examination of the outbreak of epidemics in Suzhou as well as local and governmental responses; Chapter six focuses on the practice of medicine in Suzhou, the emergence of *yi* as a specialized function and the development of the fields of specialties.

Notes

[1] Richard von Glahn, *The Sinister Way: The Divine and the Demonic in Chinese Religious Culture* (Berkeley: University of California Press, 2004).

[2] Prasenjit Duara, "Superscribing Symbols: The Myth of Guandi, Chinese God of War," in *Journal of Asian Studies* 47.4: 778–95.

[3]Kim Taylor 's book *Chinese Medicine in Early Communist China, 1945–1963: Medicine of Revolution* (London: Routledge Curzon, 2004) explores the construction of TCM in early communist China. Bridie Andrews, "Traditional Chinese Medicine as Invented Tradition," in *Bulletin of the British Association for Chinese Studies* 6 (1995), pp.6–15. Elisbeth Hsu, *The Transmission of Chinese Medicine* (Cambridge: Cambridge University Press, 1999), pp.6–8. See also Ralph Crozier, *Traditional Medicine in Modern China; Science, Nationalism, and the Tensions of Cultural Change* (Cambridge: Harvard University Press, 1968), pp. 151–209.

[4] The name literally means "south of the river" (Yangzi river) and includes Suzhou, Songjiang, Changzhou, Jiaxing, and Huzhou as its core administrative regions

[5] The fluctuation of silver imports into China has been well-researched by William Atwell, though there is continued debate over whether decline of silver imports contributed to the demise of the Ming dynasty. For a summary of the arguments, see William S. Atwell, "Another Look at Silver Imports into China, ca 1635–1644" in *Journal of World History* 16.4 (2005): 467–489. See also Richard von Glahn, *Fountain of Fortune: Money and Monetary Policy in China, 1000–1700* (Berkeley: University of California Press, 1996), especially Chapter Seven that deals with the "monetary crisis."

[6] Although this was felt more keenly in the hinterland in the north than in the major commercial centers of the Yangzi. Von Glahn, *Fountain of Fortune*, p. 221.

[7] Ramon H. Myers and Yeh-chien Wang have looked into economic developments from mid-seventeenth through eighteenth-century China. They pointed out the expansion of cash crops and handicraft industries in the Jiangnan region. See "Ramon H. Myers and Yeh-chien Wang, "Economic Developments, 1644–1800" in *The Cambridge History of China*, v.9, Part One: *The Ch'ing Empire to 1800*, ed. by Dennis Twitchett and John K. Fairbank (Cambridge: Cambridge University Press, 2002), pp. 563–645.

[8] Kenneth Pomeranz as quoted in Ramon H. Myers and Yeh-chien Wang, "Economic Developments," p 574.

[9] Benjamin A. Elman, *From Philosophy to Philology: Intellectual and Social Aspects of Change in Late Imperial China* (Cambridge: Council on East Asian studies, Harvard University, 1990), p. 12.

[10] Yuanhe was created in 1724 by a division of Changzhou.

[11] The professionalization of medicine has been a major theme in the field of the history of medicine, although the focus has been on the Western medical tradition and the emergence of licensing laws, formal medical instruction, and growing political and social power of physicians in creating a professional identity. The institutional and intellectual traditions in traditional China were fundamentally different from those in the West, thus even though there was a developing sense of professional identity, the strategies that were employed were different.

[12] Susan Mann, *The Talented Women of the Zhang Family* (Berkeley: University of California Press, 2007),p. 57.

[13] Donald Harper, *Early Chinese Medical Literature: The Mawangdui Medical Manuscripts* (London: Kegan Paul International, 1998), pp. 4–5.

[14] Vivienne Lo, *The Influence of Western Han Nurturing Life Literature on the Development of Acumoxa Therapy* (PhD Dissertation, London University, 1998).

[15] Sivin, 2002, p. 44.

[16] Unschuld, 2003, gives a detailed discussion on the concepts of *yin/yang*, five agents, and subcategorizations, see especially pp. 83–124.

[17] Asaf Goldschmidt, *The Evolution of Chinese Medicine: Song Dynasty, 960–1200* (London: Roudledge, Taylor & Francis Group, 2009).

[18] Marta Hanson,"Robust Northerners and Delicate Southerners: The Nineteenth-Century Invention of a Southern Medical Tradition," in *Positions* 6.3 (Winter 1998): 515–550. Also *Inventing a Tradition in Chinese Medicine: From Universal Canon to Local Medical Knowledge in South China, the Seventeenth to the Nineteenth Century.* (PhD Dissertation, University of Pennsylvania, 1997

[19] *Hippocratic Writings*, ed. by G.E.R. Lloyd, translated by J. Chadwick and W.N. Mann (London: Penguin Books, 1983), p.262.

[20] *Huangdi neijing suwen 4*. Translation text taken from Ilza Veith, *The Yellow Emperor's Classic of Internal Medicine*, new edition (Berkeley: University of California Press, 1966), p. 111.

[21] This is most effectively reflected in comparative studies. See Nathan Sivin and Geoffrey Lloyd, *The Way and The Word: Science and Medicine in Early China and Greece* (New Haven: Yale University Press, 2002) and Shigehisa Kuriyama, *The Expressiveness of the Body and the Divergence of Greek and Chinese Medicine* (New York: Zone Books, 1999).

[22] Charles Rosenberg, "Introduction," in Charles Rosenberg and Janet Golden ed. *Framing Disease: Studies in Cultural History* (New Brunswick: Rutgers University Press, 1997), p. xiv.

[23] Eliot Freidson, *Profession of Medicine: A Study of the Sociology of Applied Knowledge* (New York: Dodd, Mead & Company, 1970), p. xviii.

[24] Michel Foucault, *Power/Knowledge: Selected Interviews and other writings 1972–1977*, ed. by Colin Gordon, translated by Colin Gordon, Leo Marshall, John Mepham, Kate Soper (New York: Pantheon Books, 1977), p. 176.

[25] Michel Foucault, *The Birth of the Clinic: An Archaeology of Perception*, translated by A.M. Sheridan Smith (New York: Vintage Books, 1973), p. 196.

[26] Ibid.

[27] For example M. Jeanne Peterson, *The Medical Profession in Mid-Victorian London* (Berkeley: University of California Press, 1978) traces the changing character of medical

prestige and the evolution of medical men's authority in nineteenth-century England. Guenter Risse's study of the Royal Infirmary of Edinburgh in the eighteenth century—*Hospital Life in Enlightenment Scotland* (Cambridge: Cambridge University Press, 1986) shows how the mercantilist ideology contributed to the medicalization of society and brought questions of health and disease to the forefront of social policy. See also Charles Rosenberg, *The Care of Strangers: The Rise of America's Hospital System* (New York: Basic Books, 1987); and also Morris Vogel, *The Invention of the Modern Hospital, Boston: 1870–1930* (Chicago: University of Chicago Press, 1980).

28 See Eliot Freidson, *Profession of Medicine: A Study of the Sociology of Applied Knowledge* (New York: Dodd, Mead & Company, 1970). Freidson looks at the emergence of the medical profession as it displaced law and the ministry from their once dominant positions. Also Robert Dingwall and Philip Lewis ed., *The Sociology of the Professions: Lawyers, Doctors, and Others* (London: The MacMillan Press, 1983).

29 For example Nathan Sivin believes the *ruyi* "did not constitute a profession as many sociologists define the word. They were not organized, did not think of themselves as a group, and could not set or enforce common standards of medical education, skill, or compensation." *Traditional Medicine in Contemporary China* (Ann Arbor: The University of Michigan Press, 1987), p. 21.

30 *Kaozheng* literally means searching for evidence, the emphasis was on the rigorous analysis and collection of impartial evidence from ancient documents and texts.

31 Benjamin A. Elman, *From Philosophy to Philology: Intellectual and Social Aspects of Change in Late Imperial China* (Cambridge: Harvard University Press, 1984), pp. 96–100.

32 John W. Dardess, *Confucianism and Autocracy: Professional Elites in the Founding of the Ming Dynasty* (Berkeley: University of California Press, 1983).

33 Ogawa, Teizo ed., *History of the Professionalization of Medicine.* Proceedings of the 3rd International Symposium on the Comparative History of Medicine—East and West. October 8–14, 1978. Susono-shi, Shizuoka, Japan.

34 Paul Unschuld, " The Physician in Imperial China, Medical Ethics and Malpractice Legislation," in *History of the Professionalization of Medicine*, edited by Teizo Ogawa. Proceedings of the 3rd International Symposium on the Comparative History of Medicine—East and West. October 8–14, 1978. Susono-shi, Shizuoka, Japan, pp. 91–115, quote on p. 91.

35 Ralph Croizier, Traditional Medicine in Modern China: Science, Nationalism, and the Tensions of Cultural Change (Cambridge: Harvard University Press, 1968), p.34.

36 Manfred Porkert, "Intellectual and Social Impulses Behind the Evolution of Traditional Chinese Medicine" in *Asian Medical Systems*, ed. by Charles Leslie (Berkeley: University of California Press, 1976), p. 70.

37 Joseph Needham, "Medicine and Chinese Culture" in *Clerks and Craftsmen in China and the West* (Cambridge: Cambridge University Press, 1970), p. 265.

38 For a discussion of the transmission of medical knowledge see Yamada Keiji "Igaku no denju" (The transmission of medicine" in *Yorunaku tori* (Tokyo: Iwanami shoten, 1990) pp. 55–96.

39 The field owes much to the groundbreaking work of Joseph Needham and Lu Gwei-djen, members of the "High Ancestors" in the broader field of the history of science, technology, and medicine in East Asia,[39] but the focus of Needham and Lu had mostly revolved around the "Needham Question": why China was overtaken by the West in science and technology despite her early supremacy in these fields. Today this question is no longer considered conducive to understanding scientific and technological developments in China. Much of this shift can be attributed to a "second generation" of scholars, includ-

ing Sakade Yoshinobu, Yamada Keiji and Nathan Sivin, who approached Chinese science and medicine by situating them within China's cultural and political milieu.[39]

[40] Henry E. Sigerist, "The Social History of Medicine" in *Henry E. Sigerist on the History of Medicine*, Felix Marti-Ibanez, ed. (New York: M. D. , 1960), pp. 25–33.

[41] The terms "High Ancestor" and "second generation" come from the 12th International Conference on the History of Science in East Asia (ICHSEA), held July 14–18, 2008 at the Johns Hopkins University in Baltimore, USA. The Conference was dedicated as a tribute to the "second generation."

[42] Robert Hymes, "Not Quite Gentlemen? Doctors in Sung and Yuan," in *Chinese Science*, 8 (1987): 9–76.

[43] T.J. Hinrichs, *The Medical Transforming of Governance and Southern Customs in Song Dynasty China, 960–1279* (PhD Dissertation, Harvard University, 2003)

[44] Charlotte Furth, *A Flourishing Yin: Gender in China's Medical History: 960-1665* (Berkeley: University of California Press, 1999).

[45] Angela Leung Ki-Chi, "Organized Medicine in Ming—Qing China: State and Private Medical Institutions in the Lower Yangzi Region," in *Late Imperial China* 8.1 (1987): 134–165. On an earlier period, "Medical Learning from the Song to the Ming," in *The Song-Yuan-Ming Transition in Chinese History*, ed. by Paul Jakov Smith and Richard von Glahn (Cambridge: Harvard University Press, 2003): 374–398.

[46] Yili Wu, "The Bamboo Grove Monastery and Popular Gynecology in Qing China," in *Late Imperial China* 21.1 (June 2000): 41–76. Also *Transmitted Secrets: The Doctors of the Lower Yangzi Region and Popular Gynecology in Late Imperial China* (PhD Dissertation, Yale University, 1998).

[47] Marta Hanson,"Robust Northerners and Delicate Southerners" and *Inventing a Tradition in Chinese Medicine: From Universal Canon to Local Medical Knowledge in South China, the Seventeenth to the Nineteenth Century.* (PhD Dissertation, University of Pennsylvania, 1997).

[48] Joanna Grant, *A Chinese Physician: Wang Ji and the 'Stone Mountain Medical Case Histories* (London: Routledge Curzon, 2003).

[49] In the field of Western medicine, this question has created strain between "medical historians," doctors who used their expertise to interpret medical changes while focusing on the great achievements and breakthroughs in medicine, and the "historians of medicine," scholars trained in historical analysis who looked at medicine through its social context.[49] Some scholars have bemoaned the disappearance of medicine in the study of its history: the proliferation of "medical history without medicine." They argued for a reorientation of the field. See for example Lloyd G. Stevenson, "A Second Opinion," *Bulletin of the History of Medicine*, 54 (1980): 134–40; and [Leonard Wilson], "Medical History Without Medicine," *Journal of the History of Medicine*, 35 (1980):5–7.

[50] As quoted in [50] Benjamin A. Elman, *On Their Own Terms: Science in China, 1550–1900* (Cambridge: Harvard University Press, 2005), p. xxx.

[51] Benjamin A. Elman, *On Their Own Terms: Science in China, 1550–1900* (Cambridge: Harvard University Press, 2005)

[52] Ibid., pp. xxx–xxxxi.

[53] There have been efforts to shift the direction, for example the China Institute for History of Medicine and Medical Literature of the China Academy of Traditional Chinese Medicine in Beijing and the journal *Zhonghua yishi zazhi* (Chinese Journal of Medical History) publish articles that explore intellectual and social aspects of medical development. On the other hand, we find scholars actively engaged in the social and cultural analysis of the history of medicine, for example the works of Angela Ki-Chi Leung, Chu Ping-yi, Chang

Chia-feng, and Hsiung Ping-chen, all attempt to bring social and cultural analysis to their studies of medicine.

[54] There are exceptions for example Volker Scheid, who is trained as a physician also.

PART ONE

The Medical Landscape in Late Imperial Jiangnan

CHAPTER ONE

The "Confucianization" of Medicine: The Idea of the *Ruyi* (Confucian Physician) in Late Imperial China

> *buwei liangxiang, ji wei liang yi*
> If one cannot become a good prime minister,
> one should become a good physician.
>
> Fan Zhongyan (989–1052)[1]

THIS aphorism by Song scholar-official and Suzhou native Fan Zhongyan became a cliché in medical treatises and scholarly writings from the Song dynasty onwards. Its ubiquitous use by scholars and physicians alike testifies to a recognized connection between medicine and the intellectual tradition that was dominated by the *ru*, and an acceptance of medicine as a possible alternative to civil service. [2] This change in attitude towards medicine reflected changes in the background of physicians and the ascendancy of the notion of *ruyi* (Confucian physicians).[3] The community of physicians that emerged was intricately related to that of the community of scholars and book publishing in late imperial China. Labeling and categorization of physicians according to their own moral and intellectual criteria was part of an effort by the emerging community of physicians to establish boundaries and criteria of inclusion and exclusion. This process emphasized the moral ethics of medicine, while discussions of the medical classic contributed to Confucian physicians awareness to establish legitimacy.[4] This effort was largely conducted through literary debates among physicians and scholars. The effort on part of the Confucian physicians to elevate their status intensified in late imperial times as competition became keen especially in the Jiangnan region. These Confucian physicians not only wanted to establish their superiority among physicians, but because medicine was also a practical profession, they needed to attract patients. Since there were no state issued licenses to legitimize their positions and testify to their effectiveness as healers, they had to rely on other strategies. This Chapter explores the efforts by Confucian physicians to establish their moral and intellectual authority over other practicing physicians, especially the hereditary physicians, by claiming the authority of an orthodoxy in classical medicine based on a textual tradition, and the construction of a sage presiding over this orthodoxy. This was an effort not only to elevate their position but also prove their effectiveness as physicians. This was accomplished through two major debates: the proper interpretation of *sanshi* (three generations), and the assertion that Zhang Zhongjing was the medical sage instead of merely being one of the *sidajia* (four major schools).

The reason why these debates are significant is that there is an inherent tension embodied within the term *ruyi* (Confucian physicians). Were they scholars or were they artisans? The common background in the training of Confucian classics enabled many physicians to share a language with the scholars. There was constant interaction between the classical medical tradition and the classical intellectual tradition. Medical knowledge had always been considered as necessary for the complete education of a Confucian scholar. Confucian morality and ethics were often used as power leverage in the attempt to delineate a boundary for acceptable behavior.

The elite physicians dominated medical discourse in late imperial Suzhou and created a lively forum for medical discussion. At the same time, a growing sense of themselves as a distinct group emerged. The elite physicians had always attempted to exert moral and ideological control over the practice of medicine through an image of the ideal physician and a linkage to the Confucian conceptions of virtue. This not only allowed them to exert symbolic and ideological control over the profession, but at the same time elevated their status.

The Ideal Physician: The Question of *Sanshi* (Three Generations)

Both hereditary physicians and Confucian physicians wanted to distinguish themselves from the folk healers. The emphasis on benevolence and a sense of moral superiority enabled them to elevate themselves above the others. Within this elite group of physicians, debates over the necessary character and knowledge enabled them to demarcate boundaries of inclusion and exclusion. They established criteria of legitimacy based upon the classical tradition. The literary networks provided them with the opportunity to foster a sense of identity among themselves, not through legislation or licensure, but through cultural and social means.

The debate here centered on the proper interpretation of a passage in the Chapter on *Quli* (Hidden rituals) in the *Liji* (Book of Rites). The passage reads "One should not take the medicine of a physician who does not come from three generations." (*yi bu sanshi, bu fu qi yao*) The question is what this "three generations" referred to. In popular interpretation, it was generally taken to mean that one should not take the prescription of someone who did not come from a family with at least three generations of practicing physicians. The term *sanshi* here thus referred to a family tradition in medical practice. It placed an emphasis on the medical knowledge and practical experience that had been passed down through generations.

Other scholars as well as some physicians, however, objected to this interpretation. They argued that it referred instead to three traditional medical classics attributed to legendary ancient sages: the *Huangdi zhenjiu* (The Yellow Emperor's Canon on Acupuncture), *Suwen maijue* (Classic of the Pulse of the Suwen),[5] and the *Shennong bencao* (The Divine Husbandman's *Materia Medica*). These three classics represented the three major traditions in traditional Chinese medicine on acupuncture, *materia medica*, and the study of the pulse.[6] Instead of experience, they pointed to the acquisition of classical knowledge as essential to the training of a physician. Scholars who subscribed to this view did not disagree on these three texts in particular. Medical knowledge was linked to book learning. The ideal physician shared with the scholars a common heritage since the Yellow Emperor and the Divine Husbandman were legendary sages who were cultural heroes of Chinese civilization.

The issue here, however, is much more than the appropriateness of text versus experience, for neither side rejected the importance of the other. Many scholars and physicians who advocated studying the medical classics also emphasized the importance of experience. I argue that this discourse, rather than reflecting a dichotomy between text and experience, was an attempt to elevate the social standing of the physicians by creating an identity that was associated with classical learning and expertise based on classical training in medicine. The attempt to create the image of a "Confucian physician," similarly, was an attempt to elevate the status of the physician from a mere artisan (*gong*) to that of a learned scholar. We will begin by looking at the annotations and commentaries made by scholars in the Han and Tang concerning the term *sanshi*.

The *Liji,* also known as the *Xiaodai liji* (Book of Rites compiled by Younger Dai), contains a collection of essays and treatises on rituals such as funerals, mourning, and sacrifices, with explanation of meanings and functions of these rituals. Later dynasties used these for their own purposes. During the Later Han, Zheng Xuan (127–200) wrote commentaries for the Five Classics, including the *Liji,* elevating its importance among the classics. Although Zheng was an Old Text scholar, he did not ignore New Text scholarship and his commentaries considered to be the synthesis of Han scholarship.

It was during the Tang dynasty that the *Liji* gained imperial patronage when scholars included it in the *Wujing zhengyi* (Correct Significances of the *Five Classics*). During the Tang, under the sponsorship of emperor Taizong, Kong Yingda and other Confucian scholars provided this collaborative annotation, incorporating the commentaries already made by Zheng Xuan and produced the *Liji zhengyi* (Correct Significances of the *Liji*) as part of the *Wujing zhengyi* (Correct Significances of the *Five Classics*). Its contribution was that, as Peter Bol has argued, "it integrated, ranked, and summarized an extensive tradition in a single set of works. It was a kind of encyclopedia of Classical studies."[7] During the Song dynasty, the *Wujing zhengyi* was incorporated into the *Shisan jing zhushu* (Commentaries and Annotations to the *Thirteen Classics*). These *Thirteen Classics* became the core of classical studies for those who aspired to an official career through the civil service examination. Evidential research scholars during the Qing dynasty still admired the *Shisan jing zhushu*[8] The annotations and commentaries by these Song and pre-Song scholars have been referred to repeatedly in the discourse on the term *sanshi* in late imperial China.

Most of the discussion on this passage of "*yi bu sanshi, bu fu qi yao*" (One should not take the medicine of a physician who does not come from three generations) in late imperial times focused on the interpretation of the term "*sanshi.*" When one reads it closely, it becomes clear that the concern expressed was not only for the experience of the physicians, but also for the safety of medicine. This latter concern is manifested more clearly in the preceding sentence which stated that, "*jun you ji yinyao cheng xian chang zhi, qing you ji yinyao zi xian chang zhi*" (When a ruler is ill and [needs to] drink medicine, the minister first tastes it; when a parent is ill and [needs to] drink medicine, the son first tastes it). Thus the filial son and loyal minister will first try the medicine before offering it to the parent or ruler. This is crucial to the understanding of Zheng Xuan's annotation of this passage in the *Liji.*

In his annotation of the *Liji* (Book of Rites), the later Han scholar Zheng Xuan did not specify any explanation for the term *sanshi* in this particular passage but noted only "*shen wu qi ye*" (caution in medicinal preparation material). When Zheng Xuan wrote this, he probably had in mind the problem of the preparation and safety of medicine. The lack of annotation on the term *sanshi* reflected that Zheng did not feel it needed additional explanations.

It was during the Tang dynasty that we first encounter a shift from the concern for the safety of medicine to that of the proper training and experience of physicians. This is reflected in the concern over the correct interpretation of the term *sanshi.* Kong Yingda et.al. in their annotation of this particular passage in the *Liji* stated that it referred to three practising generations of physicians.[9] The *Liji Zhengyi* (Correct Significances of the *Liji*) explained that,

> All people's illnesses are due to the imbalance of the *jin-xue* (tendons and blood), therefore [people] take medicine to cure them. If these medicines [are made] without caution as to the ingredients used, there will be no symptoms [to show it]. Thus it is better to guard against [the use of these medicines]. Select those who have passed on the tradition from father to son for three generations. This is caution in materials [used in] the mixing of medicinal preparations (*shenwu tiaoqi*).[10]

Kong continued to refute the contention that the term "*sanshi*" could refer to the three Classics of *Huangdi zhenjiu* (The Yellow Emperor's Canon on Acupuncture), *Sunu maijue* (Classic of the Pulse of the Sunu), and the *Shennong bencao* (The Divine Husbandman's *Materia Medica*), claiming that only electing to take the medicine of physicians who had studied these three classics was "inappropriate according to principle, and wrong in its meaning."[11]

Kong here was probably referring to Jia Gongyan, a Tang official and scholar, when he wrote this, for the latter said, "For the three generations, the first is *Huangdi zhenjiu,* the second is *Shennong bencao*, the third is *Sunu maijue*, also referred to as *Fuzi maijue* . If [a physician] does not study the books of these three generations, [one] should not take his medicine."[12] The discussion thus had shifted from the concern for the safety of medicine to that of the proper training of physicians. This attempt to lay down a textual foundation for the training of physicians reflected an attempt to challenge the authority of hereditary physicians whose power was based upon the proven efficacy of their medicine. By shifting to the knowledge and training needed, they could gain ascendancy over the hereditary physicians. However, Kong Yingda's insistence on its interpretation as three practicing generations of physicians shows that to see it as referring to the three classics was still not widely accepted.

The ascendancy of the Confucian tradition was established under Han Wudi (r. 141–87 B.C.) when he made Confucianism the state orthodoxy. But throughout the turmoil after the downfall of the Han, the political and cultural division of the country into the north and south was also reflected in scholarship where northern and southern schools developed. Kong's *Wujing zhengyi* (Correct Significances of the *Five Classics*) was "above all a sorting out of traditions of scholarship on texts fundamental to civilized life. While recognizing the diversity of past scholarship, it identified some commentaries and modes of interpretation as most authoritative and brought northern and southern traditions of interpretation together."[13]

In medicine, a similar trend can be found in the attempt to sort out the different traditions. Chao Yuanfang et. al., under imperial patronage, compiled *Zhubing yuanhou lun* (On the origins and symptoms of medical disorders). The importance of this work in medicine is sometimes compared to the *Wujing zhengyi* (Correct Significances of the *Five Classics*) within the Classics. The patronage of the imperial court in the compilation of medical texts such as *Zhubing yuanhou lun,* and the publication of therapies and formulae such as Wang Tao's *Waitai miyao* (Arcane essentials from the Imperial library) helped to consolidate the canonical tradition in medicine. It emerged as the tradition with the highest prestige. Other works that aided in systematization and consolidation of the various traditions can be represented by Sun Simao's *Qianjin yaofang* (Essential prescriptions worth a thousand).

Imperial interest and patronage of medicine heightened during the Mongol Yuan dynasty and there was an increase in elite participation in medicine during the Yuan.[14] As will be discussed in later sections, elite participation steadily increased during the Ming and Qing dynasties. Thus it was during this time that we begin to hear a more spirited discussion over the proper interpretation of the term *sanshi* (three generations). Many Ming and Qing scholars criticized Kong Yingda for confusing the meaning of this term. For example, Song Lian (1310–1381), in his *Zhen yishi Gemou xu* (Composition as a gift for physician Ge), believed that the correct interpretation of the phrase should be the three Classics.[15] During the Ming, Sheng in his *Yijing mizhi* (Secret guide to the meaning of the medical classics) first cited Song Lian on the issue of *sanshi* and adds:

> There are too many heroes and self-made man from antiquity to list them all. For example people like Li, Zhu Danxi , Hua Boren, Dai Yuanli [their skills] were all not passed on from [earlier] generations yet they had brilliant accomplishments in medical techniques, reviving those in grave danger numerous times, wrote books and established teachings, and became models for those who came after them. From the beginning I have not heard of [them] transmitting [their knowledge] from father to son. This shows that [the training of] physicians resides in the reading of books and not in the [transmission over] three generations.[16]

Similar sentiments can be found in Pan Ji’s *Yideng xuyan* (Continue burning the flame of the light of medicine) where he writes that, “For the way of medicine, [one must] ponder the profound and subtle, brightly illustrate the cleverness of the minds, and then can [one] be allowed to become [a physician], even fathers are not able to compel their sons to have these attributes.”[17]

Other scholars also contributed to the discussion. Hang Shijun (1696–1773), a noted historian and a major figure among the Han-Learning scholars,[18] traced in his *Yi sanshi shuo* (Discourse on three generations in medicine) the different interpretations for the term *sanshi*, and argued that in the *Neijing*, the term *shanggu* (high antiquity) referred to Fuxi, *zhonggu* (middle antiquity) referred to Shennong. Therefore Fuxi should be the *yishi* (first generation), and Shennong should be the *ershi* (second generation), thus *erhuang* (two emperors) in the *Neijing* referred to Fuxi and Shennong. This, he believed, was proof that during the time of the Yellow Emperor, the example of Fuxi and Shennong was already followed, and the works of both Fuxi and Shennong were already available. It was through the study and consultation of these works that he was able to establish his own legacy.[19] Hang also went on to endorse the study of the three Classics, writing:

> I am puzzled by today’s physicians. [Their] eyes do not see the books of *Ling* [*Lingshu, Su* [*Sunu maijue*, [their] ears do not hear the discourse of Que [Bian Que] and Fu [Yu Fu]. They boast saying that it is better to attend to actual cases than to study the books. But cases today are not any different from [those in] antiquity. They are narrated completely in the books. Those [physicians’] natural endowments are mediocre, [so that] even if they study they will not be able to explain, if they can explain it is difficult for them to understand...How can [the term] *yi bu sanshi* be devised for three generations of physicians![20]

However not all scholars and physicians agreed that the term *sanshi* should refer to the three classics. There were still those who believed that it referred to three generations of practicing physicians. For example Xu Chuanpei,. who wrote the essay "*Yi bu sanshi bu fu qi yao jie*" (Explanation of "One should not take the medicine of a physician who does not come from three generations") in *Gujing jingshe* (Studio for the philological exposition of the Classics),[21] returned to Zheng Xuan's annotation and focus on the safety of medicine. Xu Chuanpei believed that within the text the term *sanshi* did not refer to the three Classics but rather referred to three generations of practicing physicians. Even if this were not the case, one should also follow conventional explanations and regard one *shi* (generation) as thirty years. He also pointed out that elsewhere in other texts Zheng had already annotated *sanshi* as three generations, therefore he believed that this explanation should also apply to this passage. As to the meaning of *shen wu qi* , he writes:

> ...The Zhou official *shiyi* (Food Physician) says, 'Solid food medicinal preparations should be considered during spring time, thick soup medicinal preparations should be considered during summer time, paste medicinal preparations should be considered during fall time, decoctions should be considered during winter time.' All use the harmony of drinking and eating [with the seasons] as medicinal preparations. *Qi* is [therefore] the same as *ji* medicinal preparations). The "Bibliography of Art and Literature" Chapter of *The History of the Former Han Dynasty* says," The hundred medicines are mixed medicinal preparations.' This refers to medicines being mixed as medicinal preparations and [one can] no longer examine the categories of ingredients. These consist of varieties of herbs, tree, fruits, grains, metal, stone, animals, and insects. When they are mixed into medicinal preparations, then the ingredients cannot be known. Therefore [one] should not take it. ... Therefore the physician must [have practiced] for as long as three generations, only then can people believe their medicine is harmless, and perhaps will dare to take it. Without the passage of this long period of time then [one] should not take the medicine. This is what is meant by *shen wu qi* (caution in medicinal preparation material).[22]

Here, Xu referred to the concern for the safety of medicine that Zheng Xuan had expressed.

Although most Ming and Qing physicians and scholars focused on the term *sanshi*, there were those who commented on the issue of the safety of medicine. For example Qing scholar Zhu Cun noted Zheng's annotation of *shen wu qi*, but he differed from Xu's interpretation. Instead he believed that the phrase referred to the contention that effective curing medicinal preparations were embedded in the teachings of sages like Shennong. (Divine Husbandman).[23]

The lack of a discussion on the dangers of medicine as that brought up by Zheng Xuan's annotation and Xu's essay should not be seen as apathy towards medicinal drugs. The rich and long pharmaceutical tradition in China attests to a strong interest in the formulation of effective and safe medicinal therapies for the curing of illnesses.[24] Rather, the lack of an apparent interest highlights the spirited contention over the issue of *sanshi*, for it touched upon the very heart of the question of what constituted the characteristics of an ideal physician.

On the other hand, the interpretation of the term *sanshi* as "three generations of practicing physicians" was probably more widely accepted among the people. Many physicians and scholars also supported this interpretation. They pointed to the commentaries on the classic *Liji,* especially the annotations of Kong Yingda, to support their contention that this was the original meaning of the text.

Thus, beginning in the Tang, we have a continuing debate over the proper interpretation of the term *sanshi.* The continued interpretation of *sanshi* as these three Classics, however, is indicative of a more serious issue that concerned the scholars and physicians at the time. They were not arguing over which Classics to study, nor were they rejecting the importance of practical experience, but they were debating the proper qualifications and training for a physician. This issue becomes more interesting when one realizes that, in reality, the three Classics referred to by Song Lian and others were no longer extant.[25] What was the use, therefore, of insisting on the importance of studying these three non-existent Classics? The answer I believe, lies in the fact that, first, it defined the kind of knowledge and skill that was required to practice medicine. Second, it was an endorsement of the ideology and methodology of the transmission of medical knowledge. The latter was related to the formation of a canonical tradition in traditional Chinese medicine. This issue reveals the discourse on what constituted a competent physician, and his qualifications.

What emerged out of the discourse over the term *sanshi* was contention over both the training and qualifications of a competent physician and the kind of knowledge required. Out of the controversy two main lines of argument emerged. One argued for the importance of accumulated knowledge, especially knowledge on drugs, which could only be proven safe after being used for a long period of time. Those who endorsed *sanshi* as three generations of practicing physicians underlined the importance of this kind of practical knowledge, especially familiarity with drugs that were passed down through the generations. The other line of argument stated not only that a physician should be familiar with Classical texts, but should be broadly trained. Those who advocated studying the three Classics believed that physicians should be well-versed in the methods of diagnosis and treatment, and be familiar with the diverse range of drugs that were available. They also pointed to the need for a particular kind of person who would be qualified to become a physician, someone who was intelligent and perspicacious. This inner quality could not be passed down through the generations.

In the discussion by Xu Chuanpei on the annotation of the Han Confucian Zheng Xuan, it is clear that one of the major concerns was over the safety of drugs. Only hereditary physicians and their formulae, with generations of experience, could be trusted. Effective secret formulae were often jealously guarded and passed down from generation to generation. The monopoly on a cure ensured the continued patronage by patients, and thus a lucrative income. In particular, families of hereditary physicians who had established reputations for a certain specialty prospered. This kind of transmission undoubtedly posed a threat to those scholars-turned-physician who did not possess this knowledge. The call for studying classical texts was a way for scholar-physicians to counter the challenge of the hereditary physicians and to establish their own legitimacy. Since they could not compete with them, they were going to emphasize other qualities that were important.

Although the use of drugs had a long tradition in traditional Chinese medicine, most physicians agreed that the best physician did not use drugs but strengthened the constitution and *qi* of the individual to prevent the onset of illness. The best physician prevented the occurrence of illness with an emphasis on *yangsheng* (nourishment of life). It was generally recognized that the more potent the drugs the more poisonous they were. In the taking of drugs, therefore, one relied on those that had proven to be effective and safe. For families to have survived three generations was an indication of the efficacy and safety of the drugs that they used.

During the Tang (618–907) dynasty, Emperor Muzong consulted a *fangshi* (Daoist) in an effort to cure his illness, arousing the opposition and concern of many within the court. A man by the name of Zhang Gao presented a memorial to the throne but cautioned against arbitrarily taking drugs. In his memorial, the text on three generations in the *Liji* was cited as proof. Here Zhang Gao was appealing for the emperor to be cautious in his use of drugs and in the selection of healers.[26]

The emphasis on three generations of medical practice and experience was not without its advocates among late imperial physicians. You Tong a Qing physician, quoting the passage in *Liji*, wrote his praise for a physician, Chen, whose ancestors migrated to Suzhou during the Song dynasty and had practiced medicine for thirteen generations.[27] Popular sayings such as *san zhe gong zhi wei liang yi* (arm broken three times and [one] will know that he is a good physician), and *jiu zhe bi er cheng yi* (one becomes a physician after breaking the arm nine times) reinforced the importance of experience in the training of physicians.

Proponents of the other line of argument however believed that it was not only textual knowledge that formed the basis of the training of the physician, but also that broad training in the different aspects of acupuncture, pharmaceutics, and diagnosis was necessary. It was with this kind of training that would enable a physician to respond to the myriad cases that they would encounter. The three Classics of *Huangdi zhenjiu*, *Shennong bencao* and *Sunu maijue* represented the three major traditions in traditional Chinese medicine on acupuncture, *materia medica*, and the study of the pulse. Sheng Yin (1375–1441) claimed that studying the work on acupuncture was for *qubing* (expelling illnesses), studying the *Bencao* enabled one to *bianyao* (distinguish drugs), and the *Maijing* was for the purpose of *chazheng* (investigate symptoms).[28]

Pulse diagnosis was of particular importance in traditional Chinese medicine and emphasis on the pulse appeared in early classics. There were also significant developments in methods of diagnosis throughout the centuries, and, by late imperial times, Lin Zhihan advocated four methods of diagnosis: *wang* (visual observation), *wen* (listening and smelling) , *wen* (questioning), *qie* (palpation).[29] Pulse diagnosis was part of the method of palpation and was one of the most important. It had a long tradition and there were detailed descriptions of the twenty-eight types of pulses.

Therapy and treatment in traditional Chinese medicine involved a plethora of techniques. The purpose of therapy was first to strengthen the body's own *qi* (vital energy) and then to drive away the pathogenic elements that were causing the illness. In traditional medicine, therapy involves, among other methods, acupuncture, moxibustion, drugs, massage, and exorcisms. Acupuncture had traditionally been an important method of curing illnesses and was still popular during the Ming and Qing dynasties despite being abolished in the Imperial Medical Academy in 1822.[30] However it seemed to have lost its preeminent position when more physicians came to prefer the use of *tangyao* (decoctions).[31]

The most important method of therapy was undoubtedly the use of healing drugs which were derived from animals, plants, and minerals. The *materia medica* that has been attributed to Shennong (The Divine Husbandman) was probably compiled during the period of the Later Han (25–220 AD). A major effort at systematization took place during the Ming by physician Li Shizhen (1518–1655). He compiled the *Bencao gangmu* (Compendium of *materia medica*) in 1696. This work and its successor,

Bencao gangmu shiyi (Compendium of *materia medica: supplement*) became the most authoritative texts on pharmaceutics.

Those who advocated the interpretation of *sanshi* as three Classics were attempting to refocus attention on the textual tradition in medicine and the necessity of being well-versed in the three traditions of diagnosis, treatment, and *materia medica.* Only a thorough understanding of these three aspects would allow the physician to prescribe the drugs and treatments necessary to cure the patient. This was to counter the trend, perceived by many, in which hereditary physician relied too much upon the use of secret formulae (*mifang*) passed down within the family. There were also physicians who relied upon books of formulae to treat illnesses without understanding the nature of the illnesses. These physicians therefore did not possess the skills and knowledge required to properly treat patients.

In his admonishment to the sons of hereditary physicians who came to study under him, Zhang Zhicong cautioned them by saying that

> If [you] only hold on to formulae that are handed down, thinking that they have been passed from generation to generation, how different is this from selecting a horse based upon a picture? For Heaven has the *qi* of four seasons, Earth has the differences in five directions. For the hundred illnesses of man, there are many changes and illusions. Just take the case of *shanghan*, there can be three hundred and eighty-nine methods [to treat it], can one stick to the handed-down formula, and [still] thoroughly change and respond to illnesses of the seasons?[32]

Zhang was arguing that by merely following traditions and formulae handed down within the family, the hereditary physicians could not respond to particular conditions of the seasons and the individual physical constitutions of the patients. Training in the classical texts provided the physician with the necessary knowledge and ability to respond to these diverse conditions.

Zhang's writings also provide a glimpse into what could be considered the realm of private teachings in medicine. Regarding the above quoted section, it was said that he made these comments because among his students there were many who came from a hereditary background. In his *Lushan yichao* (Medical notes from Lushan), the preface mentioned that this was a collection of lecture notes from the *jiangtang* (lecture hall). [33]

The qualifications of the competent physician thus also included the ability to *biantong* (change and accommodate) and respond to different seasons and conditions. Merely relying on secret knowledge, often embodied in the secret formulae passed down from previous generations, was insufficient.

For this kind of knowledge was inadequate in treating the myriad diseases of the different seasons.

Zhang Zhicong, however, did not object to knowledge that was passed down within the family. He believed rather, that if they could also study the Classics, then this would be the ideal. He ended by quoting the Song Confucian Cheng Yi, saying, "A physician who does not study, even if he becomes [like] Cang, or Bian , ultimately belongs to the class of artisans, and is not a scholar-gentleman."[34]

The issue therefore was not just to study the classics, but *dushu* (study of books), a sentiment expressed by Sheng Yin as well when he admonished that the term *sanshi* should refer to the classics. The modes of transmission of medical knowledge underwent changes as printing made medical books more accessible and the popular dissemination of medical knowledge easier.[35] Although Sheng Yin, Zhang Zhicong and others did not specify what books to study in order to cultivate the necessary qualities of an ideal physician, i.e., one who was intelligent and perspicacious, and possessing the ability to *biantong* (change and accommodate) when faced with different circumstances, one needed to possess the qualities of a scholar and the knowledge of a physician.

The admonition of Zhang to his students was a reflection of his image of the ideal physician: the *ruyi* (Confucian physician). Many hereditary physicians were apparently also heeding the call to create the image of the ideal physician, as evidenced by the fact that they also attended Zhang Zhicong's lectures. The idea of the *ruyi* therefore was embraced not just by the scholar-turned-physicians, but by some hereditary physicians as well.

Central to the question of the proper interpretation of the term *sanshi* were issues of legitimacy. The creation of a canonical tradition in medicine gradually elevated the position of the scholar-physicians, leading to the creation of the ideal image of physicians: that of a Confucian physician. Scholars and physicians intended to create social and cultural boundaries with their ideal image of a physician. The image that was created was a physician who possessed not only medical knowledge, but also moral character and intelligence. These were qualities that many claimed could never be passed down from father to son, but had to be cultivated through the study of classical texts.

The Qing (1644–1911) scholar Zhu Cun declared in "On medicine as a gift for Zhao Linan, that "As a son, one cannot be ignorant of medicine, and medicine cannot be practiced by non-Confucians."[36] There are two meanings implicit in this sentence. The first is that knowledge of medicine was not the monopoly of the physician, but considered essential for any filial son, and filial piety was considered as one of the essential virtues of an ideal Confucian. Second, that knowledge of Confucian classics and possession of the moral character and intelligence of a Confucian were a prerequisites for the practice of medicine. Therefore medical knowledge was closely associated with learnedness and character. Zhu was arguing for forging a close connection between the Confucian scholar and medicine. This was the image of the *ruyi* (Confucian physician).

The process of the formation of a canonical tradition in medicine beginning in the first century B.C. established competition with the hereditary physicians. Sivin pointed out in his study on Chunyu Yị (also known as Cang Gong) that "The master physician was expected to choose intellectually and morally fit disciples and prepare them to receive the canons."[37] In this form of transmission, the disciple was to prepare himself ritually to receive the canons, and the significance of this is in the continuity of texts that are attributed to the legendary sages. It was believed that through the study of these texts one could gain insight into the wisdom of the ancient sages's medical practice. This pattern of transmission was not restricted to medicine, but can be found in other fields such as mathematics and permeated all Confucian book learning.[38]

Yamada Keiji studied the social formation of medical groups in early China and believes that the formation of schools originated with groups of wandering physicians. Based on the *Hanshu* (History of the Han dynasty), Yamada lists three major schools within medicine which formed from the end of the Warring States period to the early Han: School of Huangdi, School of Bian Que, and School of Master Bai. He does not mean however that Bian Que or Huangdi were the founders of these schools, but that they represented the blending of the teachings passed down through his followers and the ideas of the Yin-Yang school. The School of Huangdi probably took shape during the early Han when Huanglao influences were particularly strong, and, as a result, Huangdi was honored as the founder. With the formation of different schools of thought, the methods of transmission also changed. Formerly the physicians who settled in one place usually passed on their knowledge from father to son. With the wandering physicians, it became transmitted from teacher to disciple, just as occurred with Chunyu Yi. Yamada believes that the passage in the *Liji* reflected a distrust of this latter form of transmission. The assassination of Bian Que perhaps was a reflection of the deep division amongst the different groups of physicians.[39]

The continued reference to these ancient texts even though they were of no pragmatic value in late imperial times should also be seen in light of the development the *sanhuang* (Three Emperors) as the progenitors of the medical tradition—Fuxi, Shennong, and Huangdi. The attribution of canonical texts to legendary emperors in antiquity, and in particular to the aforementioned Three Emperors was a process that began in the Han with the compilation of the major canonical texts. However, the official establishment of the Three Emperors as the progenitors of the medical tradition began with the Yuan (1274–1368) dynasty when physicians were included in the *sanhuang miao* (Temple of the Three Emperors). It was in 1295 that Emperor Yuan Chengzong ordered the erection of temples for the Three Emperors in the local districts. For a detailed discussion on the *sanhuang miao* see Chapter Two.

The Ming scholar Song Lian, in his *Zhen yishi Gemou xu* (Composition as a gift for physician Ge), claimed that to become a physician, one had to be able to "think and ponder the profound and subtle, manifest intelligence of the mind" before one could even study medicine. These qualities, he argued, could not be passed down through the generations but had to be cultivated through a process of learning.[40] Song Lian also cited the examples of two physicians, physician Yan, who came from three generations of physicians, and physician Zhu, who was the first in his family to become a physician. The latter's family had engaged in the study of the classics for several generations before Zhu took up medicine. The former, physician Yan, often misdiagnosed cases and his patients were invariably later cured by Zhu. Song Lian lamented that many people chose a physician only because he came from a family of physicians, but did not inquire into whether he was familiar with the medical classics.[41] To strengthen their argument, these scholars and physicians referred to the famous physicians in ancient China, pointing out that they did not come from families of physicians.

Qing scholar Liang Zhangju ridiculed the interpretation of the passage in the *Liji* as three generations. This was unacceptable because, he argued, one then could not even take the medicine of physicians who came from only two generations. Furthermore, he said, none of the famous physicians in the past or the present came from three generations of physicians.[42]

Shi Lize also said that," According to my humble opinion, among those who are called the divine physicians (*shenyi*) of antiquity, there are none like Bian Que and Cang Gong. Yet the art of Bian Que was received from Changsang Jun, and the art of Cang Gong was transmitted from Gong Cheng Yang Qing . From the beginning I have never heard of them transmitting [their knowledge] through generations. As for people such as Li Dongyuan, Zhu Danxi, Hua Boren, all were courageous heroes who advanced themselves. Therefore [we] know that [to be] a physician resides in the study of the three classics, and it is not based on the three generations from the father and grandfather."[43]

The formation of a canonical tradition in medicine favored the scholar-physicians, but from all indications, it was still the hereditary physicians who dominated. This trend continued into late imperial times, and thus the lament of Song Lian that many people chose a physician only because he came from a family of physicians, and did not bother to inquire into whether he was familiar with the medical classics or not.[44]

The disagreement surrounding the proper interpretation of the term *sanshi* can be seen as part of a greater effort by physicians and scholars to delineate boundaries of acceptance into the practice of medicine in the context of intense competition. After all, if *sanshi* referred to a family tradition, then the elite scholars who wanted to earn their livings in medicine would be at a distinct disadvantage in soliciting patients and in establishing their legitimacy.

Physicians in traditional China were generally classified as artisans, and their biographies can be found in the *yishu* (artisan) sections of the official dynastic histories. Beginning in the Song, there was an increasing effort to forge a link between the Confucian tradition and medicine. In the section on Confucian physicians in the *Gujin tushu jicheng* (Collection of works past and present), Zhao Conggu commented, "I have heard that a Confucian understands propriety and righteousness, a physician understands injury and welfare. Not cultivating propriety and righteousness is like obscuring the teachings of Confucius and Mencius; not distinguishing between injury and welfare is jeopardizing the lives of the people. How can Confucianism and medicine be taken lightly? How can Confucianism and medicine be separated?"[45] Thus the inseparability of the essence of Confucianism with the practice of medicine was emphasized.

We have also seen the explicit declaration of the affinity between Confucianism and medical practice by Zhu Cun. The concept of the Confucian physician had a two-fold function. First it enabled aspiring Confucians to maintain their moral and educational superiority. It also allowed them to put the idea of benevolence into practice, i.e. express ideal Confucian values through real action. Secondly it enabled the physician to elevate the status of the group as a whole in society.

The status of medicine and medical practitioners was not only the concern of the Confucian physicians, but of physicians such as Wang Shixiong, whose family included salt officials and physicians and who also endorsed the emphasis on studying the classics. He likened the way of medicine to the way of the immortals (*xiandao*), where there was a long interval before a special person came along and truly grasped the essence of medicine. He believed it would be foolish to ignore this person because his forefathers were not practicing physicians. Wang therefore believed *sanshi* should be translated as three Classics.[46]

Wang also quoted the admonition of famous physician Ye Gui (1666–1745) to his sons before he died, warning "[m]edicine is not to be taken lightly. One must be endowed with intelligence, and have studied ten thousand books, before one can use the technique to benefit the world...my descendants should not speak of medicine lightly..." Wang asked "Should not those who rely on the reputations of their grandfathers and fathers take heed of this!"[47]

The creation of the image of the ideal Confucian physician allowed the elite to elevate the status of physicians by linking it to Confucian values, and at the same time counter the seeming popularity of the hereditary physicians. It was this process of negotiating boundaries and criteria that eventually contributed to the process of professionalization of medicine in late imperial times.As both Yamada Keiji and Nathan Sivin pointed out, even as early as the Han there were already tension within medicine between the hereditary physicians, who transmitted medical knowledge through the family, and the scholar-physicians, who emphasized the transmission of texts to worthy disciples. There was a gradual shift in the process of transmission from within the family to that of texts. But as the cases of Zhang Zhicong and Gao Shishi showed, hereditary physicians were also participating in the process of learning through texts. We can discern two main reasons for this. The first is the prestige that was attached to the canonical texts. Even though most patients preferred hereditary physicians, knowledge of texts endowed them with a kind of symbolic power which elevated their social standing. Secondly, the texts that they studied did not just include the classical texts, but a wide variety of medical works. These undoubtedly helped in broadening their training. In late imperial China, there was a flourishing publishing industry and book trade, especially in the Jiangnan area. In medicine, there were voluminous publications of medical treatises, medical primers, and a proliferation of various genres of medical publications. For example, the works published by Jiangsu physicians under the *shanghan* (Cold Damage disorder) category increased from 1 in the Yuan, to 27 in the Ming, to 183 in the Qing; in *neike* (internal disorders) from 10 in the Yuan, to 121 in the Ming, and 336 in the Qing.[48] An increase in these works reflected a growing interest in these fields in medicine, and a market for them. Increased publication contributed to the dissemination of medical knowledge and the creation of a network of literary communication among the scholars and physicians, especially in the Jiangnan region. There was also a dramatic increase in the number of works on the history of medicine (*yishi*). In Jiangsu, it increased from 18 in the Ming to 160 in the Qing.[49] Heightened interest in the history of medicine reflected an increasing attempt to establish a lineage for medicine. Lineage was traced to the medical classics attributed to the ancients sages of the Yellow Emperor and the Divine Husbandman. It established the authority and legitimacy of the canonical tradition and challenged the authority of the hereditary physicians. The discourse in the interpretation of *sanshi* in the *Liji* was part of the effort to affirm the lineage of texts and reject the sole reliance on a family lineage. The increase in medical publications corresponded to an increase in the number of physicians. Compared to the Song and Yuan times, the number of physicians in Jiangsu province increased dramatically.[50] This led not only to competition for legitimacy and the effort to establish the canonical tradition as the most prestigious, but there were also efforts to impose greater conformity and standards in the practice of medicine and in the training of physicians. Xu Dachun, for example, was dissatisfied with what he perceived to be an influx of failed examination candidates into the medical profession. These people, he believed, were only looking for a way to make a living. He thus advocated the establishment of medical examinations to ensure that those who practiced medicine knew the words of the sages and treated illnesses in accordance with the knowledge passed down since antiquity.[51]Here, Xu Dachun was more specific than many of his contemporaries in advocating a system of evaluation for the practice of medicine. This was especially important in light of the fact that unlike in Europe, the Chinese state did not have licensing laws or criteria for regulating the practice of medicine in general. Without any formal system of evaluation, the different groups of physicians competed in their claims for legitimacy. The formation of this community of can be attributed to an increased participation by the elite in medicine. Medical practitioners in Suzhou were a diverse group, including scholars turned physician, hereditary physicians, and a variety of folk practitioners. It was however, an influx of elites that was the most remarkable. This increase can be attributed to population growth in the region which translated into keener competition for the civil service examinations, as each province was allocated a set quota for passing the examinations. The Japanese scholar Miyazaki Ichisada estimated that in late imperial China, approximately one in three thousand was lucky enough to pass the series of examinations and obtain the highest level of *jinshi* (Metropolitan Graduate).[52] As a result, the biographies of many a physician testify to an abandoned quest for an official career. Medicine was an acceptable alternative not only because of the potentially lucrative income, but because medicine also fulfilled the Confucian ideal of benevolence. The changing composition of the community of medical practitioners brought to the forefront issues of legitimacy and boundaries of admission. This was played out not in the conflicts over licensing laws as had occurred in Europe, but in debates over the proper form of medical knowledge necessary for a physician.

Economic developments in the lower Yangzi region also contributed to more fluidity among the different social classes. One finds many officials engaged in commercial activities that were traditionally frowned upon by the elite. But it was also the common intellectual background which enabled many of the physicians to share a common language with the scholars. The diverse group of medical practitioners often employed the same symbolic vocabulary to bolster their positions in their competition for legitimacy. It is within this context that we see the attempts to construct a professional identity by the physicians.

The most striking difference from their European counterparts was that, for aspiring Confucian physicians, their status in society was tied to their literary talents, and that there was a lack of an institutional framework to protect and enhance their monopoly and privileges as healers. In other words, the late imperial physician could not look toward the state to protect his rights to practice medicine, nor could he rely on the state to grant him legitimacy.

At a time when one could practice medicine simply by hanging up a symbolic gourd (*hulu*), the influx of elite into medicine in late imperial China created much tension among the physicians. Thus the discourse on the term *sanshi* was not merely an exercise in the interpretation of classical texts, but also part of an attempt to establish legitimacy by the elite. However, even in their attempts to establish supremacy over the hereditary physicians, the scholar-physicians did not deny the importance of experience and the need for specialized knowledge. It was the accumulation of experiences that allowed for the development of fields such as *yangkẹ* (wounds and skin infections) and *erke* (pediatrics), fields that were often mentioned in the biographies of physicians. There was a general recognition among physicians of the importance of specialized knowledge and that different illnesses should be treated by physicians who were knowledgeable in that particular field. Chapter Six discusses specialized fields in more detail.

For patients who had to choose from the wide variety of physicians, the important criterion was reputation. This emphasis on the efficacy of treatments remained a major criterion of judgment in traditional Chinese medicine. Even with the increasingly close ties to the classical tradition and the creation of an ideal Confucian endowed with intellect and cleverness, efficacy continued to play an important role in the validation of the status of a physician. The creation of a textual lineage closely associated with the Confucian tradition gave them symbolic power, but it was still their skills and reputation as healers that brought patients to them.

In this diverse field of medicine, the state did not regulate medical practice.[53] In addition, as seen from Zhu's writing, medicine was not the monopoly of physicians but considered an essential attribute of a filial son. Therefore, the question of who had legitimacy over the practice of medicine was debated by both practitioners and scholars. The discussion involved not just the proper character for an ideal physician, but also what made a good physician. It is within this context that we find a growing discourse on the identity of the physician in late imperial times and on the notion of what exactly constituted the ideal physician (*yi*). This discourse was dominated by the physicians in the classical tradition.[54] Their efforts reflected attempts to create an ideal image of the physician—that of a Confucian physician (*ruyi*).

Construction of a Medical Sage: Zhang Zhongjing and S*idajia* (Four Major Schools)

Another issue that generated passionate discussions among physicians and scholars revolved around the status of Zhang Zhongjing, author of the famed *Shanghanlun*. Was he one of the Four Major Schools? Or did he reign above them all as *yisheng* (medical sage)? The attempt to elevate the status of Zhang Zhongjing to that of a sage reflected the continued effort to create an orthodoxy that matched the lineage of the *ru* (Confucian) tradition.

The work *Shanghanlun* did not gain widespread dissemination or recognition until it underwent re-editing and re-arrangement by Wang Shuhe during the Jin dynasty (265–420). Up till then, the work was passed on mainly through private transmission. This led Sun Simiao of the Tang dynasty to lament that "the practitioners of the south (*jiangnan*)[55] secretly transmitted Zhongjing's formulae and did not disseminate them."[56] There were thus competing centers of medical practice. *Shanghan lun* gained wider transmission and importance under the Song government's sponsorship of the publication of medical works. It was edited by Sun Qi and Lin Yi and this edition came to be known as the *Songben* (Song edition). This text was also part of a required curriculum in the Imperial Medical Academy, further elevating its importance. The development of movable type print made printed texts more accessible and medical texts, including that of *Shanghanlun,* were widely printed and disseminated.

Scholars generally see the Song (960–1279), Jin (1115–1234), and Yuan (1264–1368) periods as the starting point for the emergence of medical lineages in traditional Chinese medicine. In the section on medicine in the *Siku quanshu zongmu tiyao* (An Abstract on the Index to the Complete works of the Four Divisions), it is noted that schools (*menhu*) in Confucianism began to emerge in the Song, whereas schools in medicine started in the Jin and Yuan periods.[57]

More specifically, in the Ming there emerged the notion of the *Jin Yuan Sidajia* (The Four Major Schools of the Jin-Yuan Period)—Zhang , Liu , Li, Zhu. It is generally agreed that the latter three refer to Liu Wansu (1110/20?–1200), Li Gao (1180–1251), and Zhu Zhenheng (1281–1358). The point of contention among the Ming and Qing physicians was who "Zhang" referred to. Ming physicians such as Li Zhongzi (1588–1655) and Zhang Jiebin (1563–1640) believed that it referred to Zhang Ji (Zhang Zhongjing) of the Later Han.

Li Zhongzi in his *Yizong Bidu*[58] (An Essential Reading on Medicine) commented on the Four Major Schools and writes:

> Distinguished people from ancient times, unless they each have their own ideas and share the same foundation, their works will not be perpetuated. Even if they are perpetuated they will not necessarily be highly regarded. For Zhongjing Zhang Ji, Shouzhen Liu Yuan[sic] Wansu, Dongyuan, Li Gao, and Danxi Zhu Zhenheng, what they have propagated are the most important in the medical community, they are called the Four Major Schools because they each established their own school. They explained the important meanings of the *Neijing* and expounded on what people previously have not covered and do not hinder or follow each other. They complement and explain each other. Zhongjing wrote *Shanghan Fanglun* which states that the *liuqi* of *feng, han, shu, re, shi, zao* can all harm people, but *hanxie* is the *qi* which is killing and can harm people the most. Also the changes in the *liujing*[59] is difficult to understand and the *yin* and the *yang* are similar and thus easy to be misled. If the formula is a fraction off it kills people faster than the blade of a knife. Therefore [Zhongjing] set down three hundred and ninety-seven methods and one hundred and thirteen formulae in order to supplement what was not completed in the *Neijing*, and he established his own school.[60]

Another Ming physician Wang Lun [61] in his *Mingyi zazhu* [62] (Collection of Miscellaneous Experiences of Ming Physicians) commented:

> People ask: of the various works of Zhongjing, Dongyuan, Hejiang, Danxi, which one is better? Which one should one study as the primary? Answer: it is better to

> concentrate on the *Neijing* as the primary and broadly read the four masters. This way there will be no disadvantages. *Neijing* is to medicine is just like the six classics is to the way of the Confucians, it is all encompassing. The works of the four masters are just like *Xue, Yong, Yu, and Meng*[63] are the ladders to the six classics; not one can be left out. For the works of the four masters, there is initially no superior or inferior, but that they each expound on one meaning.[64]

Both Li Zhongzi and Wang Lun have placed the work of Zhang Zhongjing of the Later Han together with that of the three physicians from the Jin and Yuan periods. Although they recognize the usefulness of Zhang Zhongjing's work, it represented only another school of thought which was incomplete without taking into consideration the developments in the Jin and Yuan periods.

This provoked a strong reaction from Qing physicians such as Xu Dachun (1693–1771), Zhang Jingtao, and Lu Yitian (1802–1865) who believe that Zhang Zhongjing should not be put on the same level as the other three. Xu commented that

> The state of medicine is indeed gloomy. The people of Ming had a view that there are four major schools, meaning the four people Zhang Zhongjing, Liu Hejian, Li Dongyuan, and Zhu Danxi, and claim them to be the great masters of medicine for a thousand antiquity. This is truly ignorant preposterous talk. Master Zhongjing is the sage who has epitomized a thousand antiquities. He is like Confucius for the Confucians. Hejiang and Dongyuan are but a side study, and Danxi only considered the words of the various schools and made selections to discard or to keep, and opened the door for students to study conveniently and easily. These are what the common people call famous physicians. Comparing the three men to Zhongjing, they cannot even hope to be his one ten thousandth. Yet they are placed alongside and spoken of together, does this not make one roar with laughter. For example people like Bian Que, Cang Gong, Wang Shuhe, Sun Simiao do truly have disciples succeeding, but they also only formed one school. For example in the Confucian school, those various scholars from the Han and Tang can definitely not be put on the same level as Confucius. Even less so these three men. As for the talents of these three people, although Liu venerated the *Neijing*, but he in reality has not been able to get its essence. Zhu is ordinary, easy and simple, but he has not been able to grasp the origins. As for Dongyuan, he holds on to the theory of the *piwei*, using only the method of uplifting [energy] and using fragrant and dry [remedies]. His ideas are partial and methods arbitrary, and he misles later learners. He is the exact opposite of Zhongjing. Later generations are quite taken with his ideas, and this is because men in the world have not even been able to know medicine even in their dreams, that is why they are misled. Even more alarming is that some think that since Zhongjing has written the book *Shanghanlun*, and think that it specializes in shanghan, and *Jingui Yaolue* cannot be used to cure illnesses. This kind of talk is even more ridiculous. I am not trying to deliberately ridicule the three men, but if this idea becomes prevalent then the world would only know the remnants of these three people, and will not search deeply for the knowledge of Zhongjing. Then the doctrines which

> Zhongjing have continued on from early sages will be in decline every day from now on. Ten thousand generations in the world will be misled. The damage is not light, so it should be vigorously corrected.[65]

Xu Dachun's sentiments were echoed by Lu Yitian in his *Lenglu yihua bupian*[66] (Supplement to Lenglu's Medical Discourses) in which he asserted that Zhongjing should be considered as a sage (*sheng*) in medicine, and that none who came after him has been able to attain the same kind of achievements. He believed that the 'Zhang' refers instead to Zhang Congzheng (1156–1228) because Hejian, Dairen (Zhang Congzheng), and Dongyuan were the three schools which Danxi refered to in his discussions. Similarly, Zhang Jingtao in his *Aitang yihua*[67] (Medical Discourses of Aitang) hailed Zhang Zhongjing as the founding father of a hundred generations of medicine and disputed that the other three could measure up to his accomplishments.

Not all Qing physicians subscribed to Xu Dachun's view. For example Li Zhiyun in his preface to Ye Gui's (1667–1746) *Linzheng zhinan yian* (Collection of Medical Cases for A Guide to Diagnosis) lists Hejian, Dongyuan, Danxi, and Zhang Zhongjing as the four major schools.[68] Therefore, we find many skeptical comments concerning the late Ming's physicians's classification of the various schools. Xu Yong, a Jiangnan physician in the early nineteenth century, has argued in his essays on the four major schools and on Li Zhongzi's *Yizong bidu* (An Essential Reading on Medicine) that people should read the classics such as the *Neijing* and *Shanghanlun* rather than Li Zhongzi, suggesting its title be changed to *bubidu* (non-essential reading).[69]

The classical medical tradition had often been influenced by developments in the dominant intellectual tradition where we find the adoption of a similar kind of language in the two traditions. For example Zhu Zhenheng in his *Gezhi yulun* made use of the idea of 'gewu zhizhi' that was prevalent in neo-Confucianist discourses at the time. The *xiantian, houtian* theories of the Song philosopher Shao Yong could also be found in medicine, for example, to refer to the *shen* as the basis of the *xiantian* and the *pi* as the basis of the *houtian.* There was constant interaction between the classical medical tradition and the classical intellectual tradition, and medical knowledge was always considered necessary for the education of a Confucian scholar.

However the classical medical tradition itself was a dynamic entity and reacted to its own internal developments. In the late Ming and Qing periods, we have already seen that many of the physicians were concerned with the systematization and classification of medical knowledge as well as with the authenticity and validity of some of the texts. It was during this period also, that partly in reaction to these activities, there emerged a group of physicians who espoused different methods of classification of illnesses and treatment. This trend developed also in part due to the accumulation of medical experiences and the effects of several large scale epidemics during this period.[70] In the next Chapter we will examine the *sanhuang miao* (Temple of the Three Emperors) and the efforts by the state to endorse a medical orthodoxy that claimed a lineage from the collective cultural heroes of China.

Notes

[1]This motto probably came from a story of Fan Zhongyan. Wu Ceng, *Nenggai zhai manlu* (Leisure Notes from the Nenggai Studio), 13:4a–b in *Mohai jinhu* (Golden Vase in the Sea of Ink) (Shanghai: Boguzhai, 1921).

[2] Robert Hymes has discussed the career strategies of Fuzhou elite during the Song and Yüan, pointing out that the increase in the number of physicians during the Yüan was brought about by fewer teaching opportunities due to the abolition of the civil service examination. This had not been the case in the Song when there was a demand for teachers in the local areas. Robert Hymes, "Not Quite Gentlemen? Doctors in Sung and Yuan," in *Chinese Science*, 8 (1987): 9–76.

[3] I translate *ru* as Confucian, using the term in its wider meaning of belonging to a particular group who are literate and share the language and values of the classical tradition associated with Confucius

[4] Chu Ping-yi pointed out in a study of Confucian physicians from the Song to the Ming that although linkage to Confucianism enabled the Confucian physicians to separate themselves from the other practicing physicians, it ultimately did not provide them with the necessary recognition as literati. Chu Ping-yi, "Song, Ming zhi ji de yishi yu ruyi" (Narrations of Histories of Medicine from the Song to the Ming and the Rise of the Confucian physician) in *The Bulletin of the Institute of History and Philology, Academia Sinica*, vol. 77, Part 3 (2006): 401–449.

[5] Instead of *Suwen maijue* (Classic of the Pulse of the Suwen), some scholars referred to *Sunu maijue* (Classic of the Pulse of the *Sunu*). The latter probably followed the annotation of the *Liji* by Kong Yingda during the Tang dynasty.

[6] The inclusion of the acupuncture text here is interesting for, in late imperial times, acupuncture was often regarded as less than an ideal form of treatment. In a study of medical practices in the novel *Jinpingmei*, Christopher Cullen points out that it was never prescribed by the *taiyi* group, but was considered the domain of physicians with low status. Christopher Cullen, "Patient and Healers in Late Imperial China: Evidence from *Jinpingmei*," *History of Science*, vol. 31 (1993): 99–105. However we must note that here it was the ancient text of the Yellow Emperor that is cited, not a reference to the practice of acupuncture. It is therefore the authority of the text that is important here.

[7] Peter K. Bol, "*This Culture of Ours": Intellectual Transitions in T'ang and Sung China* (Stanford: Stanford University Press, 1992), p. 79.

[8] For example the Xuehai tang (Sea of Learning Hall) in Canton during the Qing reprinted the *Shisan jing zhushu* and continued it with the publication of *Huangqing jingjie* (Qing exegesis of the Classics), which was chiefly concerned with evidential scholarship. See

Benjamin A. Elman, *From Philosophy to Philology: Intellectual and Social Aspects of Change in Late Imperial China* (Cambridge: Harvard University Press, 1984), p. 90.

[9] *Shisan jing zhushu* (Annotations and commentaries to the Thirteen Classics), ed. by Ruan Yuan ,1815 reprint of Song edition. (Shanghai: Jinzhang tushuju, 1926), *Liji*5, *Quli xia*, p. 6b.

[10] Ibid.

[11] *Shisan jing zhushu* , p. 6b.

[12] Quoted in Tamba no Mototane compiled, *Zhongguo yiji kao* (A Study of Chinese medical texts), published 1826 (Beijing: Renmin weisheng chubanshe, 1983), p. 187.

[13] Peter K. Bol, *"This Culture of Ours,"* p. 79.

[14] See Robert Hymes, "Not Quite Gentlemen? Doctors in Sung and Yuan," in *Chinese Science* 8 (1987): 9–76.

[15] Song Lian, in his *Zhen yishi Gemou xu* (Composition as a gift for physician Ge), in *Song Wenxian gong quanji* (Complete essays of Mr. Song Wenxian) *Sibu beiyao* edition, *juan* 44 (Taibei: Zhonghua shuju, 1965), v.116.

[16] Sheng Yin, "*Yi bu sanshi bian*" ('An Analysis of [the saying] "A physician doesn't come from three generations."') in Yijing *mizhi* (Secret guide to the medical classics), preface 1418 (Jiangsu: Jiangsu kexue jishu chubanshe, 1984), pp. 35–36.

[17] Pan Ji's *Yideng xuyan* (Continuing burning the flame of the light of medicine), first printing 1652, current volume based on 1652 edition, with 1664, 1742 editions as references. This work originated in the Song as *Siyan maijue* (Four character rhyme on the pulse) by Cui Jiayan It was edited in the Ming by Li Yan. In the Qing, Pan Ji added commentaries and formulae to become *Yideng xuyan* (Beijing: Renmin weisheng chubanshe, 1988), p524.

[18] Most of his writings on medicine were collected in *Daogu tang wenji* (Collected essays of the Daogu Hall).

[19] Hang Shijun , *Yi sanshi shuo* (Discourse on three generations in medicine) in *Daogu tang wenji* (Collected essays of the Daogu Hall), p. 10b, 13a–b in *Daogu tang quanji* (Complete collection of the Daogu Hall) (Shanghai: Shaoye shanfang, n.d.).

[20] Ibid., p. 14a.

[21] Xu Chuanpei , "*Yi bu sanshi bu fu qi yao jie*" (Explanation on "One should not take the medicine of a physician who does not come from three generations") in *Gujing jingshe* (Studio for the philological exposition of the Classics), 6 *ji*, *juan* 8, pp. 137a–b. My thanks to Ryan S. Boynton for obtaining this article for me.

[22] Ibid.

[23] Zhu Cun, "Medical Discourse: A Gift for Zhao Linan," p. 19a.

[24] See for example, Paul Unschuld, *Medicine in China: A history of pharmaceutics* (Berkeley: University of California Press, 1986).

[25] Tamba no Mototane compiled, *Zhongguo yiji kao*, p. 187. Apparently in an attempt to address this question, some later scholars replaced the *Sunu maijue* with *Neijing Suwen* (basic questions of the Inner Canon), and replaced the *Huangdi zhenjing* with *Neijing lingshu* (Divine pivot of the Inner Canon).

[26] *Xin jiaoben xin Tangshu* (New edited version of the New History of the Tang), *juan* 118, *liechuan* 43, p. 4289.

[27] You Tong "*Shudetang ji* (Record of the Hall of Establishing Virtue) in *Wujun fuli zhi* (Annals of Wu prefecture Fuli district), *juan* 21, pp. 36a–37a.

[28] Sheng Yin, "*Yi bu sanshi bian*" ('An Analysis of [the saying] "A Physician doesn't come from three generations."'), p. 35.

[29] Lin Zhihan, *Sizhen juewei* (Selection of the subtleties of the four methods of examination), 1723 (Tianjin: Tianjin kexue jishu chubanshe, 1993). Lin's work represented the growing sophistication of methods of diagnosis in late imperial China. For a discussion of these methods see Nathan Sivin's discussion and translation on the four methods of examination in his *Traditional Medicine in Contemporary China: A Partial Translation of 'Revised Outline of Chinese Medicine* (1972) (Ann Arbor: Center for Chinese Studies, University of Michigan, 1987), pp. 173–177, 291–327.

[30] This abolition is noted in Ren Xigeng, "*Tai yiyuan zhi* "(An annal of the Imperial Medical Academy) in *Qingdai zhanggu zhuilu*(A collection of historical records of the Qing dynasty), edited by Zhou Kangxie (Hong Kong: Congwen shudian, 1971), p. 169.

[31] See for example Qing physician Xu Dachun and his lament on the lack of prestige of acupuncture and moxibustion, and the deterioration of the skills of the physicians in this method of treatment in *Zhenjiu shichuan lun* (Discussion on the loss of transmission of acupuncture and moxibustion) in *Yixue yuanliu lun* (Topical discussions on the history of medicine), preface 1757 (Beijing: Zhongguo shudian, 1987), pp. 2b–3a.

[32] Zhang Zhicong, *Lushan tang leibian* (Classified argumentation from the Lushan studio), published 1670, in *Lushan tang leibian* (Classified argumentation from the Lushan studio) and Gao Shichi, *Yixue zhenchuan* (The true transmission of medicine) (Beijing: Renmin weisheng chubanshe, 1983), p49.

[33] Zhang Zhicong and Gao Shichi, *Lushan yichao* (Medical notes from Lushan), preface by Zhang Zhicong dated 1699 (Taibei: Tianyi chubanshe, 1973). It is unclear whether these were lectures by Zhang or Gao.

[34] Ibid. Cang and Bian referred to Cang Gong and Bian Que, two famous physicians in ancient China.

[35] For a discussion of the transmission and dissemination of medical knowledge between the 12th and 15th centuries, see Wu Yiyi, "A Medical Line of Many Masters: A Prosopographical Study of Liu Wansu and Hist Disciples from the Jin to the Early Ming," in *Chinese Science* 11 (1993–94): 36–65.

[36] Zhu Cun, "An essay on medicine as a gift for Zhao Linan" in *Xiaowanjuan zhai wengao*(Drafts from the Small Studio of the Myriad Scrolls) 1885 edition, *juan* 6, p. 18b. Zhu Cun had achieved the status of *jinshi* (presented scholar) in the civil service examination during the reign of the Jiaqing emperor (1796–1820).

[37] Nathan Sivin, "Text and experience in classical Chinese medicine," in *Knowledge and the Scholarly Medical* Traditions, ed Don Bates (Cambridge: Cambridge University Press, 1995), p.183.

[38] Ibid., p. 187–188.

[39] Yamada Keiji, *Yigaku no denju* (The transmission of medicine) in *Yoru naku tori* (Tokyo: Iwanami shoten, 1990), pp.66–68.

[40] Song Lian, in his *Zhen yishi Gemou xu* (Composition as a gift for physician Ge)

[41] Ibid.

[42] Liang Zhangju, *Langji congtan*, *juan* 8 in *Liangshi biji* (Notes of Mr. Liang) , 1918 edition

[43] Quoted in Pan Ji, *Yideng xuyan* (Continuing the flame of the light of medicine), p. 524.

[44] Song Lian, *Zhen yishi Gemou xu* (Composition as a gift for physician Ge)

[45] Zhao Conggu, *Ruyi pian* (On Confucian physicians) in *Yibu zonglun* (Complete discourse on medicine) under *Yishu dian* (Record on artisans), *Gujin tushu jicheng* (Collection of works past and present)

[46] Wang Shixiong *Qianzhai yihua* (Medical discourse from the Qianzhai studio), preface 1853 in *Zhongguo yixue dacheng* (A Comprehensive collection of Chinese medical works) v.6 (Zhangsha: Yuelu shushe chubanshe, 1990), pp. 830–853.

[47] Ibid., p. 853.

[48] For more details see 'Table of Medical Works by Jiangsu Physicians" in Chapter Four

[49] Ibid.

[50] See Chen Daojin and Xue Weitao ed., *Jiangsu lidai yiren zhi* (Collection of Jiangsu physicians from successive dynasties) (Jiangsu: Jiangsu kexue jishu chubanshe, 1985).

[51] Xu Dachun, *Kaoshi yixue lun*(On examinations in medicine) in *Yixue yuanliu lun* (Topical discussions on the history of medicine),pp. 14a–b.

[52] Miyazaki Ichisada, *Kakyo:Chûgoku no shiken jigoku*. (The Civil Service Examinations: China's Examination Hell) 1963 first edition, (Tokyo: Chûô kôronsha, , 1986), p.199.

[53] Although there were imperial medical academies and local medical academies , these had no authority over the practice of medicine.

[54] I have dealt with the formation of the classical tradition more extensively in "Patronizing Medicine: The *Sanhuang miao* (Temple of the Three Emperors) in Late Imperial China" (paper presented at the annual meeting of the American Historical Association, New York City, January 2–5, 1997)

[55] The *jiangnan* that is referred to here by Sun Simiao is a reference to Henan, the native place of Zhang.

[56] Sun Simiao, *Qianjin yaofang*

[57] *Siqu Quanshu congmu tiyao*, v. 2 (Shanghai: Shangwuin shuguan, 1933), p. 85.

[58] Li Zhongzi, *Yizong bidu*, preface 1637, v. 1 (Beijing: Zhongguo shudian, 1987), pp. 2a–4a

[59] Here *liujing* (six channels) refers to *taiyang, yangming, shaoyang, taiyin, shaoyin, jueyin*. In the *Shanghanlun* the *shanghan* diseases are classified as six kinds of syndromes, each listed according to the channel involved, also taking into account the degree of involvement and the progress of the illness.

[60] Ibid., pp. 2a–2b.

[61] His exact dates are unknown but he passed the *jinshi* examination in 1484.

[62] The preface for the original work was written in 1502. It later was edited by another physician Xie Yi and published in 1549.

[63] This refers to *Daxue* (Great Learning), *Zhongyong* (Doctrine of the Mean), *Lunyu* (Analects), *Menzi* (Mencius).

[64] Wang Lun, *Mingyi zazhu*, preface 1549 (Jiangsu: Kexue jishu chubanshe, 1985), p. 1.

[65] Xu Dacun, *Yixue yuanliulun*, preface 1757 (Discourse on the Origins and Development of Medicine) in *Huixi yian* (Medical Cases of Huixi) (Beijing: Zhongguo shudian, 1987), pp. 13a–13b. This translation is somewhat different from Unschuld. For original text see Appendix II, 3.

[66] Lu Yitian, *Lenglu yihua bupian*, preface in 1897, in *Zhongguo yixue dazheng*, v. 6, p. 798.

[67] Zhang Jingtao, *Aitang yihua*, preface ? in *Zhongguo yixue dacheng*, v. 6, p.819.

[68] *Linzhen Zhinan Yian*, preface 1766, v.1 (Taibei: Guoli Gugong powuyuan, 1984), Preface, p. 1b.

[69] Xu Rong, *Sidajiabian* and *Lun `Yizong bidu'* in Tang Dalie (1792–1801) ed. *Wuyi huijiang* (Collected Discourses of Suzhou physicians) preface 1792 (Shanghai: Shanghai Kexue jishu chubanshe, 1983), pp. 108–109.

[70] For a discussion on epidemics see Helen Dunstan, "The Late Ming Epidemics: A Preliminary survey" in *Ch'ing-shih Wen-t'i* v.3, no. 3: 1–59. Also Imura Kôzen,

"Chihôshi ni Kisaiseraretaru Chûgoku Ekirei Ryakkô" in *Chûgai iji shimpô*, 1936 and 1938, in eight parts.

CHAPTER TWO

State and Medicine: The *Sanhuang miao* (Temple of the Three Emperors)

MEDICINE was an important strategic tool through which the imperial state legitimized its rule as well as extended its control. Different circumstances of state building in Europe and China meant that models of state power and criteria for measuring state authority also differed in the two cultures. The state in late imperial China not only established institutional means of control such as law and the bureaucracy, but through self-fashioning as the guardians of the people for the imperial state, moral authority was equally important. In late imperial China, the state viewed medicine not only as a technical skill, but also as a benevolent measure that fulfilled the moral obligations of the ruler, and provided a means of maintaining social order. Although, unlike in the West, the state did not set up licensing laws for regulating medicine, it was through the patronage of temples and compilation of medical works that it attempted to exert its influence over medical knowledge and the practice of medicine.

Much of this moral authority was exerted through a complicated relationship established with the elite. This relationship was by no means static or exclusively the domain of the state and elite. The example of the *sanhuang miao* (Temple of the Three Emperors) shows that this relationship was constantly moderated and occasionally usurped by the other sectors of society. The ritual space of the temple was used to assert moral and political legitimation by the state, and professional identity and legitimacy by literati physicians, but ascribed as a site of healing by the locals who in some cases installed their own symbol, the *yaowang* (Medicine King) in place of the Three Emperors.

Medicine had always been valued by the state as a technical skill. As early as the Qin dynasty (221–207 B.C.), among the works spared destruction by Qin Shihuang, the first emperor of China, were works on technical skills including medicine. Thus, although the state in traditional China did not evolve explicit institutional and legal controls over the medical profession, it was through patronage that the state tried to exert symbolic and moral control over medical practice and showed its approval of the learned tradition in medicine.

In 1570, the Vice Minister of the Board of Rites (*libu shilang)* Wang Xilie presented a memorial to the throne, arguing for the removal of the Three Emperors (Huangdi, Fuxi, and Shennong) from the temple at the Imperial Medical Academy. Instead, he proposed that officials from the Imperial medical Academy should offer sacrifices to ancient physicians only. Wang's memorial was echoed by Yin Shidan, who saw it as sacrilegious to the Three Emperors. This episode illustrates how the temple came to be the contested site where issues of legitimacy and representation were negotiated. The debate over the state's appropriation of the image of the Three Emperors as patrons of medicine reflected the growing connection between these cultural icons and the textual tradition of medicine in China.

Temples are first and foremost religious sites, but, at the same time, they embody political, social, and cultural meanings. Here we find the intersection between medical practitioners and the cultural icons of the Three Emperors embodied in a religious space. Yet this intersection was debated, embraced, and rejected, mirroring the complex relationship between physicians and state patronage of medicine.

The *sanhuang miao* (Temple of the Three Emperors), was first established in the Yuan dynasty (1264–1368) for the worshipping of the Three Emperor.[1] their assistants, and famous physicians. Yet its establishment, evolvement, and later transformation into something quite different reveal the complex web of meanings woven into this space. It is a space in which the lines of medical orthodoxy, popular medical beliefs and practices, state power and legitimacy, and local elite activism intersect.

Medicine in traditional China was a field of plurality in which there was constant interaction and shifting of boundaries between the elite and the folk traditions. The emerging textual tradition in medicine, formalized in the written texts produced between the first century B.C. and the second century A.D., traced the origins of medicine to legendary sages of Chinese civilization.[2] *Huangdi* (Yellow Emperor) and *Shennong* (Divine Husbandman) came to represent the emerging textual tradition in medicine, though there was no reference to the *sanhuang* (Three Emperors) as yet. The construction and invention of the *sanhuang* (Three Emperors)—Huangdi, Shennong, and Fuxi—as the progenitors of Chinese civilization and head of the imperial lineage during the Tang dynasty (618–907) paved the way for its association with medicine. The formal association of medicine with the *sanhuang* (Three Emperors) came during the Yuan dynasty (1264–1368) when they were ritually worshipped in the *sanhuang miao* (Temple of the Three Emperors). In 1295 Yüan Chengzong decreed the establishment of temples for worshipping the Three Emperors in the capital as well as in local districts. They were to be flanked by ten physicians and sacrifices were to be performed by an imperial physician in the capital and by medical officials in the districts.[3] Following this decree, many *sanhuang miao* were established through imperial patronage in the capital as well as in local districts through the early Ming dynasty (1368–1644).This ritual association between medicine and the Three Emperors enhanced the authority of the textual tradition, not only firmly establishing it as orthodoxy, but also granting it imperial sanction. In her research, Reiko Shinno has shown that the Yuan dynasty's patronage of medicine contributed to local elites and physicians' promotion of medical schools. She argues that the *sanhuang miao* became associated with the medical schools just as the Three Emperors were incorporated into the *Daotong* (Lineage of the Way). Thus providing the physicians with elevated status and the state with fulfillment of benevolent rule.[4]

The establishment of the *sanhuang miao* (Temple of the Three Emperors) illustrated the use of cultural strategies by the imperial state not only to consolidate control but also for the legitimation of power. The latter was especially critical for the Yüan dynasty as the Mongols attempted to impose authority over a Chinese empire. Thus it is, perhaps, not surprising that the Mongols were the first rulers to formally establish *sanhuang* temples as representations of the medical tradition. For medicine, it marked the culmination of the process of domination by the Huangdi school of thought and elevated the status of literati physicians. In traditional China, medicine has always been a heterogeneous field with a fluid relationship between the classical textual tradition of the elite and the religious healing traditions at the folk level. The creation of a medical lineage was a continuous effort to establish orthodoxy within the medical tradition, and this ritual association with the *sanhuang* represented the elevation of the status of medicine from a mere "*yishu*" (craft) to a "*xue*" (learning).

Patronage of the *sanhuang miao* by the state allowed it to extend its cultural authority over medicine, and the creation of *sanhuang miao* in local districts enabled this cultural authority to reach the local levels. It also bolstered the Huangdi tradition as the medical orthodoxy. However state patronage did not guarantee the continued acceptance of the authority of the orthodox tradition, and the meaning of the temple space in the local areas would be negotiated and transformed over the centuries. From the late Ming to the Qing, we witness its transformation from a temple of legitimacy to a temple of healing, sometimes undergoing a radical transformation with the *sanhuang* replaced by the *yaowang* (Medicine King). From the mid-Ming onwards, many of these *sanhuang miao* were either abandoned or transformed into *yaowang miao* (Temple of the Medicine King). Some of these came to be widely patronized by people in the local districts. The transformation of the *sanhuang miao* from imperially sponsored ritual temples for medicine to popular local temples of healing illustrates broader issues of interaction and exchange between the textual and the popular tradition.

The increasing popularity of *yaowang* temples from the mid-Ming onwards, and the transformation of many *sanhuang miao* into *yaowang miao* reflects the fluid boundaries between elite and popular medicine. Many of the figures worshiped in these temples were famous physicians from the past, and their growing popularity with the general public, particularly the elevation of Sun Simiao to the position of *yaowang*, reflected the acceptance of the authority of the elite tradition in medicine. However, at the same time, their deification also showed a merging with religious healing in the folk tradition.

The rise and decline of the significance of the *sanhuang miao* as representation of the orthodox tradition in medicine illustrates the close relationship between state and medicine, as well as the heterogeneous nature of traditional Chinese medicine. The transformation of many of the imperially sponsored *sanhuang miao* into locally supported and patronized *yaowang miao* during the late Ming and Qing suggests that even the prestige of state patronage was not enough to allow one school or group to monopolize medicine. The growing popularity of the *yaowang miao* indicates that local traditions and folk beliefs continued to play a major role for the majority of the people, which in turn influenced the development of medicine overall. Local elites often organized and played an active role in promoting the *yaowang* temples.

This Chapter is divided into four parts: in the first part, I examine the construction of the Three Emperors as the cultural and imperial progenitor in the Tang dynasty, and its association with medicine. The second part looks at the establishment of the *sanhuang miao* as the temple for physicians during the Yuan dynasty. This joining of medicine and the *sanhuang* was not without its controversies, and the third section traces the debates surrounding the establishment of the *sanhuang miao* in the Yuan and Ming dynasties. The discussion includes the debates over the appropriateness of physicians performing rituals for the Three Emperors. These debates reveal the inherent tensions within the arrangement and the perceived elevation of artisans to the level of literati. The last part focuses on the decline of many of these *sanhuang miao*, and the transformation of some into *yaowang miao*, which was dedicated mainly to the famous physician Sun Simiao. It shows the intersection of both notions of popular healing and elite activism.

Construction of the *sanhuang*: representation in culture, imperial lineage, and medicine

The first question that arises when examining the Three Emperors and their temples is their identity. The term *sanhuang* first appeared in *Lüshi chunqiu* (ca. 239 B.C.) and is associated with the construction of the idea of *sanhuang wudi* (Three Emperors and Five Rulers) that appeared during the turmoil of the Spring and Autumn (722–481 B.C.) and Warring States period (403–221 B.C.).[5] However the identity of the three emperors varied until the construction of the triumvirate of Huangdi, Shennong, and Fuxi during the Tang dynasty. For example, in early records such as the *Shiji* (Records of History) by Han historian Sima Qian, the term Three Emperors referred to *tianhuang, dihuang, taihuang*. The efforts to determine who exactly were the Three Emperors and the Five Rulers have been subjects of debate by scholars throughout the generations.[6] Embroiled in the differences in interpretation was conflict between the *jinwen* and *guwen* factions. The veneration of various cultural heroes such as Yao, Shun and Huangdi existed prior to the Tang.[7] However before the Tang, there were no written guidelines for offering sacrifices to former emperors.[8]

The formal worship of the *sanhuang* (Huangdi, Fuxi, Shennong) by the imperial lineage began in the Tang dynasty (618–907) when a temple was erected for *sanhuang wudi*. It was also during the Tang dynasty that there was common acceptance that they referred to Fuxi, Shennong, and Huangdi. Song scholars also accepted this configuration and it seems to have continued into the late imperial times. The question then arises, why did the Tang formalized the worship of the Three Emperors? The answer is related to the construction of the cultural heroes and sages of Chinese civilization during the Tang, which were part of a larger effort to establish what Peter Bol calls a "cultural synthesis" in the early Tang.[9] The sages were looked upon as guides for the society and government.

In view of the efforts by Tang scholars to establish a cultural lineage of venerated sages responsible for the creation of Chinese civilization, it is not surprising that the earliest attempt by the state to institute a formalized worship of the Three Emperors began in the Tang dynasty. It was in the sixth year of the Tianbao reign (747) that Emperor Xuanzong (r. 713–755) decreed the worship of the Three Emperors and Five Rulers:

> In the eleventh day of the first month of the sixth year (Tianbao), the emperor ordered that the Three Emperors and Five Rulers, who created all things and laid down the customs, always iterated [what the] tortoise shell mirrors, should be respectfully venerated. The Three Emperors: Fuxi, with Goumang as assistant; Shennong, with Zhurong as assistant; Huangdi, with Fenghou, and Limu as assistants; Five Rulers.... then select the date and establish the affairs of the temple, estimate the undertaking and set up the building. As for the musical instruments it is requested that the imperial ones be used, as for sacrifices it is requested that *shaolao* be used. Spring and fall will be the two seasons to extend sacrifices. [There will be] the placing of a Director and Vice Director. Court of Imperial sacrifices [will be responsible for] examining and correcting [the rituals]. [10]

The ritual worship of the Three Emperors thus established them as the creators of civilization in China. During the Song dynasty (960–1279) there was no indication that there were temples dedicated specifically to the worship of the Three Emperors although there were temples for Shennong and Huangdi separately, and the veneration and worship of former emperors, sages, and worthy officials continued.

Nevertheless, in the Tang and Song, there was no official linkage between medicine and the Three Emperors. However, this does not mean that there was no connection between the medical traditions and the ancient sages. On the contrary, the linkage in the medical tradition had already been forged in the Eastern Zhou and Han periods. Early medical texts illustrate this connection between medicine and the formation of the textual tradition traceable to the Three Emperors.

The earliest medical text the *Huangdi neijing*, compiled between the first century B.C. and the first century A.D., reflected the increasing dominance of the Huangdi tradition not only in medicine, but also in other fields.[11] In medicine, the formation of a learned medical tradition is related to the development of medical groups that flourished during the Eastern Zhou and early Han. Yamada Keiji believes that the formation of schools in medicine originated with contact among wandering physician groups and various intellectuals, thus stimulating their efforts to systematize medical knowledge and experience. Based on the *Hanshu* (History of the Han dynasty), Yamada listed three major schools within medicine from the end of the Warring States period to the early Han: School of Huangdi, School of Bian Que, and School of Master Bai. The School of Huangdi probably took shape during the early Han when Huanglao influences were particularly strong, and as a result Huangdi was honored as the founder[12]. The Bian Que school continued to exert an influence in medicine and is probably best represented by the work *Nanjing*. However, it was the school of Huangdi that emerged as the dominant orthodox tradition, and the the *Huangdi neijing* (Inner Canon of the Yellow Emperor) came to be regarded as the most authoritative. Although most scholars believe that this work probably was put together in the first century B.C, it appears that the current extant texts of *Suwen* and *Lingshu* did not come into existence until the mid-Tang. Other scholars such as Li Bocong believes that the School of Bian Que emerged earlier than Huangdi *xuepai* (School of Huangdi), and that it was only during the turmoil after the downfall of the Han, in the Wei, Jin and the Northern and Southern dynasties that the school of Huangdi came to emerge as dominant.[13]

Another authoritative medical classic on pharmaceutics, the *Shennong bencao*, is attributed to Shennong. The earliest connection between *materia medica* and Shennong can be found in the *Huainanzi* in which he was reported to have "tried the tastes of all herbs and [examined] the springs, whether they were sweet or bitter. Thus he informed the people of what they ought to avoid and where they could go. At that time, [Shen-nung] encountered on one day seventy [herbs, liquids, etc.] with medicinal effectiveness (*tu*)."[14]

Therefore the veneration of both Huangdi and Shennong preceded that of the formulation of the *sanhuang* triumvirate and they were selected because they already had emerged as cultural authorities in medicine. This preceded the formation of the concept of the *sanhuang* (Three Emperors), which consisted of Huangdi, Fuxi, and Shennong. There was no medical classic attributed to Fuxi, although he allegedly invented writing and created the *bagua* (eight trigrams), enabling the understanding and categorizing of various illnesses. Thus, Huangdi and Shennong were both hailed as the progenitor of medicine around the time when the Huangdi group emerged as the dominant tradition, and as the medical classics of *Huangdi neijing* and *Shennong bencaojing* were attributed to Huangdi and Shennong respectively.

By the time of the Tang dynasty, Huangdi and Shennong became formalized in the Three Emperors, and were included in the lineage of emperors and venerated as the creators of Chinese civilization. The linkage with medicine came during the Yuan dynasty when ritual worship was ordered for the Three Emperors as representation of the progenitors of medicine. This dual representation of the Three Emperors was to set the stage for the debate over the status and prestige of physicians and attempts by the state to impose control over medicine and medical practice through the creation of a lineage of physicians. There was, however, inherent tension embodied within this dual representation. The following sections will examine closely the formal establishment of the *sanhuang miao* by the Yuan dynasty and the continuing debates over the appropriateness of physicians officiating at ceremonies dedicated to the Three Emperors.

Establishment of the *sanhuang miao* in the Yuan dynasty: Ritual association between medicine and the Three Emperors

Rituals "facilitated the rectification (*cheng*), solidification (*hou*), and standardization (*t'ung*) of customs, and hence the restoration or maintenance of social harmony."[15] The Duke of Zhou was said to have ruled with the use of rituals. Confucius considered *li* (rituals) and *yi* (righteousness) the fundamental difference that separates a civilized society from a barbarian one, and the expression of *li* was predominantly in rituals. Rituals thus played a critical functional as well as a symbolic role in the state's rule. It is therefore not surprising that the Yuan dynasty would make use of rituals to legitimize their rule and restore social harmony after their conquest of China. The ritual worship of the cultural icons—the Three Emperors—by physicians was established by the Mongol rulers, even though there was no previous precedent. This is perhaps due to two factors: the Mongols did not look upon medicine as *xiaodao* (lesser way) as some Confucians, and medicine as *renshu* (benevolent craft) suited their efforts to act as a benevolent ruler to the conquered Chinese. The effect of the establishment of the *sanhuang miao* as the temple for physicians was to forge a convergence of the idea of the

Three Emperors as the progenitors of the imperial lineage and Chinese civilization, and as the progenitors of the textual medical tradition.

In 1295 Yüan Chengzong ordered the erection of temples for the Three Emperors in the local districts, flanked by their four assistants. In addition to the Three Emperors and their assistants, ten other legendary physicians, selected from various medical works, also stood along walls within the temple.[16] This inclusion of ten famous physicians within the temple mirrored the pattern at the temple for Confucius (*fuzi miao*) in which there were ten worthies (*shizhe*). Sacrifices were performed twice each year in the Spring on the third day of the third month, and in Autumn on the ninth day of the ninth month. These were officiated by an imperial physician in the capital and medical officials in the districts. The rituals performed were to be the same as those performed for Confucius.[17]

By emulating the classical tradition in their veneration of Confucius, the physicians positioned themselves as successors and guardians of an imperially recognized medical lineage, granting them a prestige similar to that of the Confucian scholars and elevated the status of medicine. This tradition of having the physicians officiate at the twice a year ceremonies for the Three Emperors at the *sanhuang miao*, and inclusion of ten famous physicians establishing the Three Emperors as the progenitors of medicine in an official capacity drew the Huangdi medical tradition under the patronage of the state. This enabled the state to extend its cultural authority over the empire through the establishment of *sanhuang miao* in local districts.

The unusual nature of this act on part of the Yüan emperor is confirmed by Yüan scholar Wu Cheng who wrote in his *Yihuang xian sanhuang miao ji* (Record of the Temple of the Three Emperors at Yihuang county):

> With medicine there is school, with school there is temple, worshipping the Three Emperors in the temple began with the exalted Yüan, this has never been [the case] before. [18]

Additionally, by ordering that the physical layout of the temple to be patterned after the Confucian temple, and the ceremonies to the Three Emperors to be the same as that of the *Kongzi miao* (Temple of Confucius), the Yüan emperor drew a symbolic parallel between the medical tradition and the Confucian tradition. This served to elevate the prestige of medicine and the status of the physicians, but as we shall see in the later discussion, also drew the ire of the scholar officials who believed the association was highly inappropriate.

It may seem strange for a foreign dynasty to ascribe formal ritual status to medicine, assigning to medicine the Three Emperors who were considered as the cultural progenitors of Chinese civilization. This is however not surprising in the fact that exactly because it was a foreign dynasty, it therefore did not consider physicians, traditionally categorized as artisans in China, as unworthy of this "honor." The Mongols had a much higher regard for physicians than the Chinese. Thus Gu Jiegang commented that Yüan Shizu's actions could be understood by the fact that he had not been exposed to the *xuntao* of traditional culture.[19] Freed from the constraints of traditional Chinese values, the Yüan did not hesitate to confer prestige upon medicine and the physicians. Another fact so influenced the Yüan was that as a foreign conquest dynasty, they needed to legitimate their rule. One method was to embrace the Dao School of classical studies and enshrining Zhou Dunyi, Cheng Hao, Cheng Yi and others[20]. They also attempted to legitimize their rule by setting themselves up as the rightful successors to the imperial lineage. Thus the performance of rituals and the offering of sacrifices to the former emperors and sages took on a particular significance for the Mongols. They resumed the worshipping of the Three Emperors in the capital, but, most importantly, they ordered the establishment of *sanhuang miao* in the provinces as well. The establishment of the Three Emperors as the progenitors of the medical traditions allowed the Mongols to present themselves as the benevolent and rightful ruler of the Chinese people, who not only rectified social and political ills, but also bodily ills.

The ritual worship of the Three Emperors: Huangdi, Shennong, and Fuxi transformed what had hitherto been a faction within the medical tradition into the orthodox group. The worshipping of the Three Emperors also enabled medicine to forge a link with the classical literary tradition as well as to impose a façade of unity in the medical tradition. Temples dedicated to the worship of deities in medicine flourished in traditional Chinese society, often each with different specialties. These deities included both legendary physicians as well as famous practicing physicians of the past. Also, it was not uncommon to have diverse regional differences in the deities worshipped or in the ways of worship. This diversity reflected the cultural diversity in China. Effective rulers of vast empire understood the nature of diversity and regional differences even while regarding cultural unity and shared values as essential. Thus in medicine, it is not surprising to find the imposition of the learned tradition in medicine to mask the diversity in medical practices. The state attempted to achieve this goal through the establishment of a system of medical schools teaching the classical medical tradition, publication of medical works and pharmaceutical formulae, provision of medical relief in times of need, and also through rituals.

However, this veneration of the Three Emperors as founders of the medical tradition did not proceed without protest. In 1299, Jin Zhao, Erudite (*guansong boshi*) of the Court of Imperial Sacrifices (*Taichang si*) dissented on grounds that the Three Emperors and their assistants, as described in the *Tang hui yao*, were revered as the creator of culture and initiator of laws and regulations, now officials are

> taking the temple of Confucius (*fuzi)* and the ten worthies (*shizhe*) [worshipped in there] as example to set up ten generations of famous physicians, and offer them sacrifices. If this is indeed carried out, [then] taking the great sages of the Three Emperors and limiting them to being the ancestors of the specialized medical traditions, and to determine the ceremonies for them [based on this connection], seems too disrespectful. [In addition], investigations into the histories also did not find any reference to the ten generations of famous physicians.[21]

Jin Zhao was thus concerned most about the lowering of the status of Confucians and also assigning too low a ritual role for Confucius. Nevertheless, despite his objection, the worshipping of the Three Emperors as the progenitors of medicine continued and formalized in the first month of 1309. Following ancient tradition, following the example in the temple for the great Confucian *wenxuan*, the god of wood was placed in the center with ten great famous physicians flanking the two sides of the temple.[22] In this way, it was said that "the order of honorable and humble, first and last, is not confused."[23]

Ritual was not the only means by which the Yüan dynasty utilized to underscored the importance of medicine and elevated the status of physicians. They also sought to establish greater control over the transmission of medicine through the Imperial Medical Academy as well as in the provinces. Yüan officials created temples not only for the ritual worship of the Three Emperors, but also as sites for lecture halls (*jiangtang*). For example the *sanhuang miao* at Jiankang, begun in the winter of 1318 and finished in the fall of the next year, included a lecture hall at the back of the main hall. Yu Ji's record of Chongren *xian*'s *sanhuang miao* and Ji'an lu's *sanhuang miao* also show that lecture halls were built when the temples were renovated.[24] This reveals the importance attached to medicine by the Mongols, and their attempts to promote practical professions. With the abolition of the civil service examinations, the number of scholars engaging in medicine increased, and more elite chose medicine as a profession during the Yüan.[25] On the other hand, the adoption of the cultural icons of Chinese civilization as the creators of the medical traditions and the patterning the temple worship on that of the Confucian temple also served to erode the prestige of the Confucians, of whom the Mongols were wary.

The call for the local districts to establish *sanhuang miao* led to the proliferation of *sanhuang miao* in local areas. From the writings of Yüan scholars Yu Ji and Wu Cheng, we not only have records of the building of these temples but also of the nature and layout as well. They also reveal to us some of the difficulties encountered, for despite imperial sponsorship, it seems that financial woes plagued some of the temples.

In *Jiankang lu sanhuang miao ji* (Record of the Temple of the Three Emperors at Jiankang Circuit),[26] Wu Cheng wrote of the rebuilding of the dilapidated *sanhuang miao.* Even as the seat of the various Circuits of Jiangnan and of the Censorate, the *sanhuang miao* at Jiangkang fell into disrepair. The original site was too small for expansion, and it was not until the acquisition of over ten *mu* of government land that they were able to rebuild. Donations came from officials as well as from physicians and the common people.[27] Similarly in *Yihuang xian sanhuang miao ji* (Record of the Temple of the Three Emperors at Yihuang county), while the temple for Confucius had undergone renovations, the *sanhuang miao* occupied only a dismal building. In 1314, the official Zi Yangshi decided to renovate the temple and apparently supplied government timber for the building. However, labor and financing apparently came from private sources.

Yu Ji aso recorded precarious financial situation and private sponsorship of the *sanhuang miao*. In his *Ji'an lu sanhuang miao tian ji* (Record of the land of the Temple of the Three Emperors at Jian Circuit) he reports that there were no funds for worship at the *sanhuang miao* and that money often had to come from the physicians. In 1336 reports indicate that one Deng Mingyuan, who had received grants of land, decided to donate half to medicine. It was the income generated from renting this land that provided financing for sacrificial ceremonies physicians's stipends.[28]

Thus, despite the decrees by Yüan emperors to establish *sanhuang miao* throughout the country, the Yüan government apparently did not allocate enough resources to sustain and maintain the temples and the offering of sacrifices. Unlike the Confucian temples which received grants of land, the *sanhuang miao* apparently were left on their own. Rebuilding and renovations depended on individual officials and on money from private sources.

This can be attributed to the fact that the Yüan rulers were interested primarily in the symbolic value of patronage for medicine.

The financial difficulties of the *sanhuang miao* as well as other temples did not escape the attention of officials, they increased allotments to the temples, including *sanhuang miao*, in 1317 above the criteria set in 1305,[29] though the effect of this increase is not clear.

Therefore it was in the Yüan that the Three Emperors became officially established as the forefathers of medicine and physicians began to officiate at the ceremonies offering sacrifices. This formation of a medical orthodoxy was closely tied to the Yüan's attempts to legitimate their rule as well as to the emerging importance of the learned tradition in medicine. It allowed the state to claim patronage of medicine and bring about a sense of unity over the diverse medical traditions. Another significant development of the *sanhuang miao* in the Yüan was its spread into the provinces. Whereas in the Tang the Three Emperors were worshipped in the capital, the Yüan ordered all provinces to construct *sanhuang miao*, thereby extending their cultural authority throughout the country.

The *Sanhuang miao* in the Ming and Debates over its Appropriateness

The fall of the Mongol dynasty and the re-establishment of a Chinese dynasty did not bring about the end of imperial patronage of the *sanhuang miao,* but it did revive concerns about the appropriateness of associating the Three Emperors with medicine. During the Ming dynasty, the Three Emperors were worshipped separately in the capital in the *diwang miao* (Temple for rulers and kings)[30] and in the *sanhuang miao.* The latter was in the Imperial Medical Academy as well as in local districts. This continued association of the Three Emperors with medicine caused considerable consternation among officials. Ming officials initiated various efforts to disassociate the Three Emperors from medicine, and presented memorials to the throne calling for the ban on physician led sacrifices to the Three Emperors. However, early Ming emperors vacillated between terminating and affirming the relationship between the Three Emperors and medicine. This vacillation in face of strong opposition from officials reflects the fact that by the Ming, the triumvir of Huangdi, Fuxi, and Shennong, had been widely accepted as the orthodox lineage for the textual medical tradition. However, beginning in the Ming dynasty, we witness a decline in state interest in maintaining cultural authority through medicine in local districts. Angela Ki Che Leung has shown that the strong involvement of the Song and Yuan states in the provision of medical care through charitable organizations, sponsorship of medical education, and the publication and dissemination of *materia medica* declined in the Ming and that this trend continued in the Qing.[31] This trend is reflected in declining state sponsorship of local *sanhuang miao*, eventually allowing for the appropriation of the space by local elite for conversion into the *yaowang miao*. This latter process will be examined later.

The reason for this decline in state interest can be understood best if the debates over the appropriateness of associating the Three Emperors with medicine are examined. It is clear from these debates that the state was ultimately concerned with establishing an orthodox imperial tradition and was more interested in establishing the Three Emperors as the creators of Chinese civilization. By continuing to patronize them in the capital but, at the same time, diminishing their presence in the provinces, they were establishing themselves as not only the legitimate successors of the imperial lineage but also as the sole undisputed protector of this cultural heritage.

The first record of the Three Emperors worshipped during the Ming was in 1368, the first year of the Hongwu emperor. The emperor decreed that the Three Emperors were to be worshipped by offering *tailao* sacrifices.[32] The next year, the four assistants: Goumang, Zhurong, Fenghou, and Limu were added and the ceremony officiated by *zhongshu canzheng* (Administration vice commissioner of the Secretariat) Cai Zhe.[33] Veneration of the Three Emperors centered on their roles in establishing the foundation of Chinese civilization. Fuxi was "the first to draw the eight trigrams, taught the people to write documents, succeeded heaven and established guidelines [for the people], and opened up the succession to true orthodoxy." Shennong was "the first to plant crops, [so that] all the people had grains to eat. He tasted a hundred herbs [and] his contribution helped ten thousand generations." Huangdi possessed "thorough changes and divine transformations, passed on [the making of] clothing and established governance and regulations."[34]

The worship of the Three Emperors by the Hongwu emperor was, therefore, to establish an honorable imperial lineage of past rulers and sages. They were not venerated as the progenitors of medicine, nor were the ten famous physicians that were part of the temple in the Yüan included. In the local districts, the *sanhuang miao* continued to function, and apparently physicians still performed the ceremonies. This inconsistency between the ceremonies performed in the capital and in the provinces seemingly went unnoticed in the first three years of the Hongwu emperor, for it was not until the fourth year of the Hongwu emperor (1371) that he expressed concern to the *zhongshu sheng* about the inappropriateness of the *sanhuang miao* in the local districts.

There were three major concerns that the emperor expressed: first, it was not officials but physicians who were officiating at ceremonies at the local districts; second, all local districts were worshipping the Three Emperors, which was considered to be a desecration of the sages; and third, Yao, Shun, and Yu were all sages and had made important contributions to China, yet later generations did not establish temples for them.[35] The Board of Rites (*libu*) was ordered to consult with various scholars and make a detailed study in order to determine the appropriateness of this practice. Thus, the Board, in consultation with the Hanlin Academy and Court of Imperial Sacrifices, reported that

> In examining previous generations of imperial rulers and worthy princes, [it is found that] since the Tang all have been sacrificed to at the imperial tombs. Tang Xuanzong established a temple for the Three Emperors and Five kings (*sanhuang wudi)* in the capital. At the time of Yüan Chengzong, then, the *sanhuang miao* were established in the *fu, zhou, and xian*, with common sacrifices during the spring and fall and used physicians to officiate. [This practice is] highly improper.[36]

As a result the Hongwu emperor ordered all local provinces and districts to end this sacrilegious practice of worshipping the Three Emperors. The Hongwu emperor was clearly concerned with constructing an orthodox lineage for the imperial throne, thus enhancing the prestige of the Ming rulers, who were successors to this lineage. His concern with establishing Yao, Shun, and Yu as part of the lineage reflected his efforts to include all illustrious sages, and appropriate the Three Emperors as the progenitors of Chinese civilization, claiming that the Three Emperors "succeeded from Heaven and set up guidelines [for the people], so as to open up the source of cultural teachings of ten thousand generations."(*jitian liji, yi kai wanshi jiaohua zi yuan*) By forbidding local districts' worship of the Three Emperors, the Hongwu emperor established the state as the only legitimate inheritor and protector of this cultural tradition. This, however, did not mean the complete disassociation between the Three Emperors and medicine. The Three Emperors continued to be worshipped in the capital in the *sanhuang miao*.

In 1536, the Shengji *dian* was established behind the Wenhua *dian*[37] for the worship of ancient physicians, and, in 1542 the Jinghui *dian* was built north of the Imperial Medical Academy. The Three Emperors and their assistants were worshipped in the Jinghui *dian* where the layout was similar to that of the Yüan *sanhuang miao.* They also included famous physicians but now the number was increased to twenty-eight, with fourteen physicians on each side. Each year a senior official (*tang shang guan*) from the Board of Rites was sent to perform the acts of ceremony, with senior officials from the Imperial Medical Academy offering the sacrifices.[38] The sacrifice they offered was that of the *shaolao*, i.e. only sheep and pig.[39]

A closer examination of the *sanhuang miao* established in 1542 in the Imperial Medical Academy reveals both a continuation with the Yüan tradition and new developments in medicine. The Three Emperors occupied the central position flanked by their four ministers. Then on the east side there were fourteen physicians: Jiudaiji, Qibo, Bogao, Guiyuqu, Yu Fu, Shaoyu, Shaoshi, Tonjun, Leigong, Ma Shihuang, Yi Yin, Bian Que, Chunyu Yi, and Zhang Ji. On the west side there were Hua Tuo, Wang Shuhe, Huangfu Mi, Ge Hong, Chao Yüanfang, Sun Simiao, Wei Cicang, Wang Bing, Qian Yi, Zhu Gong, Li Gao, Liu Wansu, Zhang Yüansu, and Zhu Yanxiu.[40] These physicians ranged from the legendary to the famous historical figures, and by incorporating these physicians in the ritual space of the *sanhuang miao,* it created an orthodox lineage in medicine that was accepted and patronized by the state.

This re-establishment of ritual worship of the Three Emperors for the physicians during the reign of the Jiajing emperor was part of a wider effort to reform rituals and ceremonies. In 1530, the Jiajing emperor undertook measures to reform the rituals concerning emperors and rulers, this effort was to *lizheng sidian* (reform sacrificial rites).[41] The collateral sacrifices to the rulers and kings at the sacrificial altar to Heaven and Earth that was established in the reign of Hongwu was now to end, and their altars moved to Wenhua *dian.* Later a separate temple was built with the same layout as the previous *diwang miao,* but with the removal of Yuan Shizu and his five officials. They moved Tang Taizong to the same room as Song Taizu, making a total of fifteen rulers and thirty-two accompanying officials.[42] It was also during this time that the Three Emperors were again ritually worshipped in the *sanhuang miao,* together with twenty-eight physicians, and with physicians presiding over the ceremonies.

The Jiajing reforms confirmed imperial patronage of the orthodox medical tradition, but dissension over the association of the Three Emperors with medicine continued after his reign, resurfacing in the succeeding reign of the

Longqing emperor. The debates that followed continued the line of argument that first, the Three Emperors were progenitors of Chinese civilization, and secondly, worship by physicians was thus sacrilegious. In 1570, the Vice Minister of the Board of Rites *(libu shilang)* Wang Xilie presented a memorial in which he argued that since the Three Emperors were already worshipped at the *diwang miao*, the worship of the Three Emperors at the Imperial Medical Academy should be abolished. Officials from the Imperial Medical Academy should instead sacrifice to ancient physicians only.[43]

Yin Shidan, echoed his memorial, blaming the presence of the Three Emperors on the officials of the Jiajing emperor, who were eager to accommodate the emperor and yet neglected to investigate fully the appropriateness of the arrangement. Yin proposed the elimination of the Three Emperors and their four assistants in the *jing hui dian*, leaving only the twenty-eight physicians in one hall, arranged according to their respective generations. In this way, it would not be a desecration of the Three Emperors, and the rituals for the former physicians would not be abandoned.[44] His request was denied.

There is little to indicate the reasons behind the denial. However, by then the relationship between the Three Emperors and medicine had been widely accepted, not just by physicians, but also by the literati, and the contribution of the sages to medicine had become part of their legacy. For example Yan Song's memorial to the Wanli emperor reflected this view. In his memorial, Yan Song underlined the contributions of the Three Emperors to medicine. He argued that their founding of the medical tradition was an integral part of their role as the progenitors of Chinese civilization, and that complete their sageness. Yan criticized Yüan's establishment of *sanhuang miao* in the provinces, believing that it tarnished *(du)* the Three Emperors. However he did not advocate the abolition of the Three Emperors in the Imperial Medical Academy. Instead, he proposed uniformity in the worship of the Three Emperors.[45]

Thus, in the capital the Ming continued with the dual worship of the Three Emperors, i.e., they were worshipped both in the Imperial Medical Academy as well as in the *diwang miao*. Despite early opposition to the association of the Three Emperors with medicine, it is apparent that by the mid-Ming onward, they were inextricably connected to the foundations of the medical tradition. Being the progenitors of medicine and contributing to the welfare of the people became an integral aspect of their sageness.

In the provinces, many of the *sanhuang miao* during the Ming can trace their development from the Yüan. However the Ming court did not encourage the construction of *sanhuang miao* in the provinces even though a temple was built for the Three Emperors in the Imperial Medical Academy. Records of *sanhuang miao* in the local gazetteers in the Ming declined drastically when compared to the Yüan, an indication not only of the lack of official interest in extending its cultural influence to the local districts through medicine, but also of the wish to only patronize the Three Emperors in the capital to confirm the ultimate cultural authority of the state.

The *Sanhuang miao* in the Qing and the Growing Popularity of the Yaowang miao

The Qing followed the Ming tradition of offering sacrifices at the Jing Huidian officiated by officials. The layout of the deities remained very much the same with some changes in the order of the twenty-eight physicians. The Minister of the Board of Rites officiated the ritual ceremonies, with offerings to the celebrated physicians on the sides performed by imperial physicians. They performed the three kneelings, nine bows, and three offerings. During the Yongzheng reign (1723–1735), the Three Emperors were offered a cow, sheep, and pig, whereas a sheep and a pig were offered to the physicians.[46] The Qing also continued with the practice of offering sacrifices to the Three Emperors as ancestors of the imperial lineage in one of the seven halls of the *Jingde chongsheng neidian* on the west side of the imperial palace.[47] The lineup of the physicians along the two sides of the temple did not necessarily follow that of the Imperial Medical Academy, and one can find different variations at local temples.

The disapproval by the Ming court of provincial worship of the Three Emperors meant the cessation of funding for the *sanhuang miao* in the local districts. This contributed to the decline of many *sanhuang miao*, but, at the same time, allowed for the transformation of this physical space into a site that could be shaped by local traditions. Medicine and healing was of important practical concern for the people, and despite imperial patronage of the Three Emperors as the progenitors of medicine, the people often worshipped figures that they considered to be effective in healing. One of these was the *yaowang* (Medicine king) who became increasingly popular throughout the country as the importance of the Three Emperors declined. This transformation of the imperially sponsored temple to one shaped by local traditions and folk medical beliefs testifies to the dynamism of local medical beliefs and traditions. This latter interacts with the orthodox medical tradition that is patronized by the state but was also independent from it at the same time. The role played by local gentry in this process of change reflects the growth of elite activism and the leadership roles that they increasingly assumed not just in medicine, but also in local and national politics. In her article, Leung has shown clearly elite participation in the provision of health care in Jiangnan during the late Ming and Qing.[48]

The origins of the idea of a *yaowang* (Medicine king) can be traced back to the Buddhist canons, but the nature and identity of *yaowang* varied over the dynasties. In his article on the origin of Chinese Medicine kings, Zheng Jinsheng pointed out that the term first appeared in Buddhist canonical translations. During the Song dynasty, people considered Wei Shanjun to be the Medicine King. In the Ming, physician Xu Chunfu in his *Gujin yitong daquan* gave Wei Cizang the title of *yaowang*. There were others who have been worshipped as the Medicine King, including the legendary physician Bian Que. But during the late Ming and Qing, Sun Simiao came to be widely accepted as the *yaowang* and was popularly worshipped at the temples for Medicine Kings, although there was little historical evidence to support this claim.[49] Sun Simiao remained popular in the folk traditions and most *yaowang* temples today worship him.

Due to the changing nature of the *sanhuang miao* in the Ming and Qing, many temples gradually came to be patronized by the medicinal herb sellers and also common people who were seeking treatment for illnesses. The success of the temples thus depended upon the perceived efficacy of the healing powers of the deities. Although efforts such as the Suzhou medical students to restore the *sanhuang miao* showed that there were attempts to re-establish the importance of the medical orthodoxy and thereby elevating the status of the physicians, temples in late imperial China increasingly came to be localized.[50]

The transformation of many *sanhuang miao* into *yaowang miao* could be seen as an acceptance of the cultural authority of the elite tradition in medicine, as many of the figures worshipped were famous physicians. However, this was not a top-down transference of influence. When we examine these *sanhuang miao* turned *yaowang miao* more closely, we find that while the authority of these physicians was accepted, they were then molded and fitted into a tradition that served the needs of the people. The deification of these physicians indicated that they were being incorporated into a tradition of religious healing that had been a popular folk tradition. Their transformation into *yaowang miao* revealed a dynamic folk medical tradition that selectively integrated the textual tradition into its practices. Many sources showed that from the mid-Ming to the Qing dynasties, some of the local *sanhuang miao* were converted into *yaowang miao*. They retained the original layout of the temple but were patronized by the locals and often became sites of active markets.

In examining the development of *sanhuang miao* in the Qing, we will focus on Suzhou. The *Minguo Wuxian zhi* gives a brief account of the history of the temple for the Three Emperors. The earliest record of the establishment of a state sponsored temple worshipping the Three Emperors was in 1305 during the Yüan dynasty. This undoubtedly was due to the imperial decree that all regions in China establish *sanhuang miao*. The temple was abolished in 1371 by the Ming Hongwu emperor when he banned *sanhuang* worship in the provinces. There was no indication in the sources that the temple was revived later and it is unclear if the building was preserved for the worship of other deities.

However, in 1689, upon the request of the local medical official to the *xunfu* (Provincial Governor) Hong Zijie, the temple was rebuilt with a *jiangtang* (lecture hall) and a *yaoju* (pharmacy) at the center.[51] Two years later the *zifu* (prefect) Lu Tenglong requested the addition of six legendary physicians and the name was changed to *yiwang miao* (Temple of the Physician Kings). It was rebuilt again in 1781 and was destroyed by a fire in 1860.[52] According to an account by a Qing scholar, Peng Shaosheng, the Temple that was built in 1689 not only to worship the Three Emperors and other legendary physicians, but it also merged with a temple originally dedicated to Yu, therefore forming the worship of the *sisheng* (four sages).[53] It is interesting to note that students of the local medical academy initiated both the 1689 and the 1781 rebuilding of the temple. As the temple gradually fell into disarray during the Qianlong reign, students raised funds among their classmates to rebuild it. It's reconstruction began in the eleventh month of 1781 and was not completed until the tenth month of the next year.

There was also a *yaowang miao* in Suzhou built in 1674. People who were engaged in the medicinal herb trade patronized this temple.[54] The birthday of the *yaowang* was usually celebrated on the twenty-eighth of the fourth month with a ceremony officiated by physicians from the local medical academy. There was said to be offerings provided at another *yaowang miao* at Lujiaxiang.[55]

There seems to have been confusion concerning the *sanhuang miao* and the *yaowang miao*. As state sponsorship declined, the *sanhuang miao* in local regions often assumed the function of healing temples, rather than legitimizing the learned medical tradition and acting as sources of medical orthodoxy. The purpose of worship thus shifted to seeking efficacy in treatment rather than perpetuating a lineage. Some of the *sanhuang miao* were also renamed *yaowang miao*. Zhang Xuecheng noted on his excursion to Beijing that there was a *sanhuang miao*, which he said was built by the medicinal herb shops (*yaosi*) and, thus, was also known as the *yaowang miao*.[56]

This lack of distinction between the Three Emperors and the Medicine King prompted Suzhou physician Kang Zuolin to clarify the issue:

> Since antiquity the Three Emperors have drawn the trigrams and distinguished between the *yin* and the *yang*, distinguished the herbs and wrote the *Bencao*, discussed illnesses and wrote down the *Neijing*. For us physicians we begin our learning with the *sanfen*, and until today still study these transmitted works. [Whether] within the Medical Academy, [or] outside in the medical schools, all honor [the Three Emperors] with the main sacrificial rites, and list the regulations. Reaching the Tang [dynasty], there was [a man] with surname Wei and name Shun, his *daohao* was Cizang who distributed medicine to aid others, people in the world all looked up to him as medicine king, [this can be] verified by the history of medicine. Thus [the time between] the medicine king and the Three Emperors was already separated by the over ten generations of Tang, Yu, Xia, Shang, Zhou, Qin, Han, Jin, and the Northern and Southern dynasties. Now there are some ignorant priests, using the statue of the medicine king, and put on grass knitted clothes, so that there is no difference with the statue of Shennong. Borrowing from the writings of the *tongshu*, saying that every year the twenth-eight day of the fourth month was the birth date of the medicine king, deluding and cheating people [in order to] solicit money, so that the vulgar common people mistakenly called the Three Emperors as medicine king, it is indeed laughable...[57]

Suzhou also had many other temples dedicated to the curing of illnesses and they played a major role in the healing practices of the common people. Officials lamented the number of *yinci* (immoral temples) where the people went in times of illness. There were also numerous attempts on part of the officials to ban them.[58] One of the most popular was the *chenghuangci* or *chenghuangmiao* where it was said that the relatives and friends of the patient could pray for their loved ones' relief.

Temples for skilled physicians were also erected. In Suzhou the temple commemorating physician: Shazhen Huigongzi, was built in the reign of the Hongxi (1425) emperor, it commemorated Ming imperial physician Sha Fuyi who served in the Imperial Medical Academy in the early Hongwu period. In 1373 there was a great epidemic in the capital area (present day Nanjing), Sha set up a bureau and saved the lives of many people.[59]

The setting up of temples with official patronage showed government concern in maintaining symbolic control over the provision of medical care in the local areas. It also competed directed with local folk traditions of healing and beliefs. This worshipping of physicians in the temples serves to emphasize the practical aspect of medicine, for these physicians were honored not so much for their moral virtue or piety, rather for their skills as physicians.

The continued participation of the state in the religious sanction of medicine and the worship of the Three Emperors served to extend the cultural influence of the state into local areas. Worshipping of the Three Emperors and the famous physicians who were included within the temple provided a way for the state to exert its moral and symbolic control over medicine.[60] However this extension of the state's cultural influence was not uncontested, and the transformation of the physical space of the *sanhuang miao* into a temple for the Medicine King reflected a setting in which the cultural authority of medicine was negotiated between the textual tradition patronized by the state and the popular traditions of healing. Confucian physicians in the Ming and the Qing increasingly claimed mastery of the textual tradition as the sole source of legitimacy, arguing for the importance of knowledge of text in the practice of medicine.[61] Yet the transformation of the *sanhuang miao* shows that they were not the only ones to have authority over the textual tradition. Popular beliefs and practices often utilize it for their own purposes. The boundary between the textual and popular traditions is thus a rather fluid one.

Notes

[1] The Three Emperors worshipped in the temple were Huangdi (Yellow Emperor), Shennong (Divine Husbandman), and Fuxi (Ox Tamer).

[2] The most authoritative early medical classics ascribed to legendary sages, Huangdi (Yellow Emperor) and Shennong (Divine Husbandman), are the *Huangdi neijing* (Inner Canon of the Yellow Emperor) and the *Shennong bencaojing* (The Canon of the Divine Husbandman). The *Huangdi neijing* is a collection of heterogeneous writings by various authors that most scholars believe was compiled sometime between the first century B.C. and the first century A.D. See for example Yamada Keiji, "Kôtei naikyô no seiritsu" (Formation of the *Huangdi neijing*) in *Shisô* 662 (1979): 94–108; Geoffrey Lloyd and Nathan Sivin, *The Way and the Word: Science and Medicine in Early China and Greece* (New Haven: Yale University Press, 2002), pp.75–76; *Huangdi neijing yanjiu dacheng* (Comprehensive Collection of the Study of the Inner Canon of the Yellow Emperor) ed. by Wang Hongtu 2 vol. (Beijing: Beijing chubanshe, 1997), chapter 1. For a study of the work in English, see Donald Keegan, *The "Huang-ti Nei-ching": The Structure of the Compilations; The Significance of the Structure* PhD Dissertation, University of California, Berkeley 1988 (Ann Arbor: University Microfilms International. 8916728). For a comprehensive study and translation of the *Shennong bencaojing,* see Paul Unschuld, *Medi-*

cine in China: A History of Pharmaceutics (Berkeley: University of California Press, 1986).

[3] Yuanshi 76, p.1902

[4] Shinno Reiko, "Medical Schools and the Temples of the Three Progenitors in Yuan China: A Case of Cross-Cultural Interactions" in *Harvard Journal of Asiatic Studies* volume 67 no. 1 (June 2007): 89–133.

[5] The idea of constructing a lineage faded in the Western Han, reviving during the late Western Han through efforts of Wang Mang, who wanted to legitimize his usurpation of the throne.

[6] There are six major configurations of the *sanhuang*. First, according to the *Hetu Sanwuli*, it refers to "tian huang, dihuang, renhuang." Second, *Shangshu Dachuan* lists "suiren, fuxi, shennong." Third, in *Baihutong sanhuang* is referred to as "fuxi, shennong, suiren," or ""fuxi, shennong, zhurong." Four, *Cunqiu Yundoushu* lists "fuxi, shennong, nuwo." Five, in the Qin, "tianhuang, dihuang, taihuang" were listed as the three emperors. Six, according to Kong Anguo, they referred to "fuxi, shennong, huangdi." Thus the later configuration of the Three Emeprors in the *sanhuang miao* were based on Kong's writings. For a detailed discussion on the development of the term *sanhuang,* see Gu Jiegang and Yang Xiangkui, "Sanhuang kao " in *Gu shi bian.* v.7. Lu Simian and Tong Shuye edited (Taibei: Ming lun chu ban she, 1971):20–282; and Meng Wentong and Miao Fenglin, "Sanhuang Wudi shuo tan yuan" in *Gu shi*_v.7 *zhong.* Lu Simian and Tong Shuye edited. (Taibei: Minglun chubanshe, 1971): 314–381.

[7] For example Qin Shihuang sacrificed to Shun and Yu, and Han emperors worshipped various former sages and worthies, including Huangdi, Zhuge Liang. Yang Jialuo, *Shitong fenlei zongzuan, juan 82, li 1* (Taibei: Dingwen shuju, 1975), pp.1a–1b.

[8] *Shitong fenlei zongzuan*, p. 1b.

[9] Bol, 1992, pp. 76–107.

[10] *Tanghuiyao, 22*, p. 430.

[11] For example, in the *Hanshu*, one can find Huangdi being used in the titles for such works as on Daoism, astronomy, medicine, and calendars. This was also the time of the appearance of Huanglao thought.

[12] Yamada, 1979; 1990: pp. 66–68. Donald J. Harper agrees with Yamada on the association of physicians with text-based traditions but disagrees with the speculation that there was the existence of medical schools. (Harper, 1998, pp. 61–62)

[13] Li Bocong, *Bian Que he Bian Que xuepai yanjiu* (A study of Bian Que and the School of Bian Que) (Shaanxi: Shaanxi kexue jishu chubanshe, 1990), pp. 96–102, 295–323.

[14] Translation of *Huai nan zi* taken from Paul Unschuld, *Medicine in China: A History of Pharmaceutics* (Berkeley: University of California press, 1986), p.11.

[15] Smith 1990, p. 283.

[16] *Yuanshi* 76, p.1902.

[17] *Yuanshi*, 76, p.1902.

[18] *Wu Wenzheng ji*, p. 7b.

[19] Gu Jiegang and Yang Shanggui, "Sanhuang kao" (A Study of the Three Emperors) In *Gu shi bian* v.7 *zhong*. Lu Simian and Tong Shuye edited. (Taibei: Ming lun chu ban she, 1971), p.258.

[20] Wilson, pp. 47–51.

[21] *Yuan dian zhang* (Regulations of the Yuan) (Beijing: Xinhua Shudian, 1990) pp.18b–19a.

[22] Confucius held the title of *Wenxuan wang*. See Thomas A. Wilson, "The Ritual Formation of Ritual Orthodoxy and the Descendants of the Sage," in *Journal of Asian Studies*, 55.3 (August 1996), p. 563.

[23] *Yuan dian zhang*, p. 19b.

[24] Yu Ji, *Dao yuan xue gu lu*. Ming edition. Sibu congkan. (Shanghai: Shangwuin chuguan, 1967), p.320 and 321.

[25] Hymes, pp. 9–76.

[26] Jiankang was located in Jiangnan, south of present day Nanjing city.

[27] Wu Cheng, *Wu Wenzheng ji* (Collected writings of Wu Wenzheng). *Ying yin Wen yuan ge Si ku quan shu*, v.1197 (Taibei: Taiwan shangwuin shuguan, 1983), p.2a.

[28] Yu Ji, p.321.

[29] *Yuan dian zhang*, pp. 20b–21b.

[30] There were five separate rooms in the *diwang miao*. The central room housed the Three Emperors (*sanhuang*); they were flanked by the Five Rulers (*wudi*) who were housed in the room to the east, and by the Three Kings (*sanwang*) in the west room. Another east room finds Han Gaozu, Emperor Han Guangwu, and Sui Wendi, and an additional west room was reserved for the worship of Tang Taizong, Song Taizu, and Yuan Shizu. Altogether there were five rooms and seventeen rulers. In 1388 thirty-seven loyal officials were added along the two sides. After a fire destroyed the *diwang miao* the same year, it was rebuilt but with Sui Wendi removed, and with Tang Taizong moved into the same room as the Han emperors, making the total number of rulers worshipped sixteen. (*Daming huidian*, 91:1433). The Three Emperors thus occupied the most prominent position in the temple, worshipped as the head of the imperial lineage. The inclusion of Yuan Shizu later led to a call by Chen Fei for the removal of the Yuan founder from the *diwang miao* (*Huangming shuzhao* 48:28a–35a).

[31] Leung, "Organized Medicine in Ming-Qing China: State and Private Medical Institutions in the Lower Yangzi Region" *Late Imperial China,* vol 8 no.1 (June 1987): pp.135–144.

[32] *Tailao* sacrifices referred to cow, sheep, pig, and according to *Liji* were for imperial sacrifices. *Shaolao* included only the sheep and pig and were used for the feudal princes. This was thus an elevation from the Tang when only *shaolao* sacrifices were used.

[33] MHY, 11: 172–173; also in MTZSL, 31:0536, 40:0802–03.

[34] MTZSL, 40: 0803.

[35] MTZSL, 63:1200.

[36] MTZSL, 63: 1200

[37] It seems that during the reign of the Jiajing emperor, in the spring of the year 1531, the rulers were moved to Wenhua dian and worshipped there, this continued the next year. The next year another temple was built at the west end of the city and the layout of the temple was the same as before, i.e. the rulers were placed in five rooms with the same arrangement. In 1545, Yuan Shizu was removed, as well as five of his officials. Emperor Taizong of the Tang moved to the same room as Song Taizu. Thus there were fifteen rulers and thirty-two officials worshipped altogether. (*Daming huidian*, 91:1433).

[38] DMHD, pp.10b–11a; MHY 11:172–173;MSZSL, 269:5307.

[39] In *Mingtaizu shilu*, 269:5307, it is said that *tailao* was used. However this is probably a mistake since in the *Da Ming hui dian* only sheep and pig are listed. (*Da Ming hui dian*, 92:11a–b).

[40] MSZSL, 269: 5307. Originally only ten physicians were included: Jiudaiji, Qibo, Bogao, Guiyuqu, Yu Fu, Shaoyu, Shaoshi, Tonjun, Leigong, and Ma Shihuang. The other eight-

een were added later, and fourteen each were arranged to line up on each side (*Mingtaizu shilu*, 269:5307). The arrangement of physicians is not explained in the texts, but they were obviously included due to their prominence in the textual tradition. This was a combination of both legendary as well as historical figures. The Qing *sanhuang miao* order of arrangement of these twenty-eight physicians is different from the Ming.

41 DMHD, 91:1433.

42 DMHD, 91:1433.

43 MMZSL 42:1034–1035; Sun Chengze, p.315.

44 Yin Shidan, "Fu shilang Wang Xilie ti zheng san huang li dian shu" in *Yin Wentong gong ji* in HMJSWB, pp. 79–82.

45 Yan Song, "Xiuzheng sanhuang sidian yi fu zu zhi yi" (A treatise on rectifying the rules on sacrificing to the Three Emperors to restore the ancestral institutions) in Chen Zilong compiled, HMJSWB, pp.17a–18b.

46 DQHD, 49:1b.

47 DQHD, 45:1a.

48 Leung, pp. 144–150. Elite activism is of course not unique only to the Ming and Qing dynasties, and they were active not only in medicine but in other aspects such as the provision of famine relief. This is especially true for the Qing dynasty. Works such as Pierre-Etienne Will's *Bureaucracy and Famine in Eighteenth-Century China* (translated by Elborg Forster, Stanford: Stanford University Press, 1990), Mary Backus Rankin, *Elite Activism and Political Transformation in China: Zhejiang Province, 1865–1911* (Stanford: Stanford University Press, 1986), and Mary Backus Rankin and Joseph W. Esherick ed., *Chinese Local Elites and Patterns of Dominance* (Berkeley: University of California Press, 1990) show the various roles local elites played in shaping local and national policies. Fuma Susumu has also demonstrated in his studies on Qing charitable organizations in the Jiangnan region the initiatives and leadership undertaken by local elites and merchants. See for example Fuma Susumu, "Shindai Songkiang ikueido no keiei jittai to chiho shakai," (Local Society and The True Conditions of Management of Qing dynasty Infant Charitable Institutions in Songjiang) *The Tôyôshi Kenkyû (The Journal of Oriental Researches*) 45.3 (Dec. 1986): 55–94.

49 Zheng Jinsheng, pp. 65–69.

50 Susan Naquin, in *Peking: Temples and City Life, 1400–1900* (Berkeley: University of California Press, 2000), gives many examples of Medicine-king temples in the city of Peking during the Ming and Qing. For example she lists twenty temples with the Medicine-king as the chief deity and twelve with him as secondary deity during the Ming and Qing (p. 37). She also examines the diverse origins of some of these temples and their changing nature.

51 *Gujin tushu jicheng*, *zhifangdian: Suzhou fu*, 677:29b.

52 *Minguo Wuxian zhi*, *tanmiaoziyu* I, 33:31a–b.

53 *Qing Peng Shaosheng Yixue Sisheng miao ji* (An essay on the Temple of the Four Sages by Qing dynasty's Pang Shaosheng), *Minguo Wuxian zhi, tanmiaoziyu* I, 33:31b.

54 (*Wumen biaoyin* (Manifest the obscure at Suzhou), *juan* 10, p.22b. It is not clear however, if this temple served as a guild for the medicinal herb traders.

55 Gu Lu, pp. 78–79.

56 Zhang Xuecheng, 22:32a.

57 Kang Zuolin, p.71).

58 *Gujin tushu jicheng*, *zifangdian*, 676:25b.

[59] *Tongzhi Suzhou fuzhi*, 37:41b.

[60] In his study on state strengthening and local power in North China in the early twentieth-century, Prasenjit Duara finds that cults such as Guandi were responsible for integrating villages to the larger society. This supported his argument for a "cultural nexus of power." *Culture, Power, and The State: Rural North China, 1900–1942* (Stanford: Stanford University Press, 1988).

[61] See Chapter One.

CHAPTER THREE

Medical Theories and the Development of the *Wenbing* School

THE most important development in medicine during the late Ming and Qing was the maturation of the *wenbing* (warm factor) theory. *Wenbing* is a broad term that encompassed a wide range of *waigan wenrebing* (externally contracted warm and hot diseases). It included both the incubating internal febrile diseases (*fuqi wenbing*) that lurked inside the body, and acute epidemics. Warm (*wen*) and hot (*re*) referred to the different degree of febrile symptoms of the patient. It thus generally referred to febrile disorders, and its chief characteristic was the appearance of fever and included both epidemic infections and non-epidemic infectious diseases.[1]

The terms *wenbing* and *wenrebing* were not new, nor was the concept of warm factor diseases. They can be found in the *Huangdi neijing* (Inner Canon of the Yellow Emperor) as well as the later medical text *Nanjing* (Canon of Difficult Questions). *Wenbing* had been considered a sub-category of *shanghan* (cold damage) based on Later Han physician Zhang Zhongjing's *Shanghanlun,* which presented a clear discussion of therapy based on symptoms, and several of his formulae became the basic standard in treating warm factor diseases. *Wenbing* was nevertheless considered a sub-category of *shanghan* (cold factor). Even though the Jin and Yuan dynasties saw greater efforts to distinguish it from the latter in causation and treatment, it did not become established as an independent and separate school until the late imperial times.

The maturation of this theory in medicine and its separation from the *shanghan* school was the result of three interconnected developments. The first was the continued theoretical developments in explaining the etiology of diseases based on observation of symptoms and experience in the efficacy of treatments. This development is also connected to an important transition in intellectual history in the Qing, that of the emerging dominance of the philological tradition. Scholars and physicians, using the methods of evidential research in the study of classical medical texts, contributed to the breakaway of the *wenbing* (warm factor) theory from the *shanghan* (cold damaged) theory. Second, the devastation and horror of a series of epidemics in the late Ming and Qing caused many physicians to re-evaluate their understanding of acute febrile diseases and search for new explanations and more effective cures. Wu Youxing and his *Wenyilun* (Treatise on Warm Factor Epidemic Disorders) represented the most thorough of these efforts. Thirdly, the economic and cultural development of the Jiangnan region led to the emergence of a center of medicine and a group of physicians who were influenced by the local environment and specificities. One of these centers in Suzhou became the site of *wenbing* scholarship. Many of the physicians participating in the development of this theory resided in the wealthy city of Suzhou, home also to many of the scholarly elite who were active participants in the intellectual transition. Physicians such as Wu Youxing, Ye Tianshi, Xue Xue, Wu Tang, and Wang Shixiong were all active in Suzhou and contributed to the development of the warm factor theory.

The maturation of the *wenbing* school therefore was a process that reflected not only evolving medical responses to illnesses, and the importance of accumulated observation and experience in medicine, but also significance in interaction with intellectual endeavors, and impact of social and economic developments. In addition, this process involved breaking out from the *shanghan* framework, facilitated by illustrating the origin of the terms *wenbing* and *wenrebing* in the *Huangdi neijing*, and tracing its intellectual lineage to the textual orthodoxy. Thus the *wenbing* school secured its theoretical separation from the *shanghan* school. Marta Hanson also sees it as an effort on part of the southern physicians to assert their separate identity from the dominant political influence from the north.[2] Susan Mann speculates that the *wenre* advocates were seen as "modern" and derided as *yongyi* by those who embraced the "traditionalist" cold-damage school.[3]

This chapter will focus on the aforementioned three inter-related developments in examining the rise of the *wenbing* school. It will show how the theoretical development of the orthodox tradition in classical medicine was closely tied to the philosophical and philological traditions, yet, as a practical craft of healing, it also generated an intimate dialogue with practitioners in the field, combining the *ru* and *yi* aspects of medicine. The legitimation of the groups of physicians who advocated the *wenbing* school therefore was based on text as well as practice derived from experiences in local specificities. The rise of the *wenbing* school provides us with a clear example of the unique tradition of classical medicine as both a scholarly exercise in the intellectual conceptualization of health and illness, and as a practical craft of healing.

Development of the Theory and Practice of the *Wenbing* school: Separation from *Shanghan*

The rise of the *wenbing* school is a complex process and I have divided it into three major phases. The first is from the formation of the *Huangdi neijing* to that of the Sui (581–618) and Tang (618–907) dynasties. This period saw the formulation of the theoretical basis and treatment courses for *wenbing,* though it was treated as part of *shanghan.* There was increasing awareness of the different causes and symptoms of *wenbing* and *shanghan*, but there were yet few attempts to extract it from a sub-category of the latter, or resolve contradictions within. The second can be traced from the Song (960–1279) through the Jin (1115–1234) and Yuan (1279–1368) dynasties. This period represented a time of tremendous intellectual flourishing due to the influx of new ideas, theoretical and therapeutic breakthroughs in the focus on the significance of heat within the body, favoring of cooling therapies, and emphasis on the nourishment of *yin.* Governmental efforts at printing and disseminating medical texts, and patronizing the classical tradition also contributed to the vibrant scene. Third, the Ming (1368–1644) and Qing (1644–1911) dynasties represented the final break with *shanghan*, the formulation of a coherent theoretical framework that explained the causes, symptoms, cure, and prevention of *wenbing.* The process reconciled one of the key contradictions in the school, enabling the establishment of an independent theory. This movement was intertwined with scholarly interest in using evidential research methods to determine the authenticity of the text *Shanghanlun.*

The origin of the term *wenbing* can be traced back to the *Huangdi neijing suwen,*[4] which not only provided the label for warm factor disorders, but also laid the basis for the three most important theoretical explanations of the disease, i.e. the notion that it was an incubating febrile disease; as a subcategory of *shanghan;* and as reference to epidemic outbreaks. The different explanation of *wenbing* reflected the diverse writings that it collected over the centuries.

The most often quoted reference in support of the first explanation is from the *Suwen* 3 "*shengqi tongtian lun*" (A Discussion on the connection of Vital Qi with Heaven) where it is said that "when injured by cold during winter, one will become ill with *wen* (warm factor) in the spring."[5] When the injury brings forth illness immediately, then it is referred to as *shanghan* (cold damage). But when the injury is incubated within the body during the winter season, emerging in the next spring, then the nature of the illness has also changed and should be regarded as *wenbing* (warm factor), relating more to internal weakness rather than external cause. This concept of incubating febrile disease within the body should be understood within the context of the importance of balancing the *yin* and *yang* within the body, and the preservation of essence and *qi.* As stated by Qi Bo in the same text," Yin stores up essence and prepares it to be used; Yang serves as protector against external danger and must therefore be strong. If Yin is not equal to Yang, then the pulse becomes weak and sickly and causes madness. If Yang is not equal to Yin, then the breaths which are contained in the five viscera will conflict with each other and the circulation ceases within the nine orifices. For this reason, the sages caused Yin and Yang to be in harmony."[6] An internal imbalance of the *yin* and *yang* created an opportunity for injury to the body to occur. This can be caused by different factors "If the wind enters the body and exhausts man's breath, then his essence will be lost and the evil influences will injure his liver. If man overeats, his muscles and pulses collapse and his bowels will be injured, resulting in bleeding piles. If man drinks too much his force of life becomes obstreperous. Those who indulge in excesses of sexual intercourse injure the force of their kidneys and hurt their loins."[7] The emphasis on wind as an agent for a cause for illness can be seen in different sections of the *Suwen.* The notions of wind and *qi* were closely related and Unschuld believes that wind and *qi* etiology developed side by side.[8] Kuriyama also points out that although wind was conceived of before *qi* and that they were sometimes used interchangeably in early classical texts, *qi* never replaced wind. Wind came to be conceived of as causes of illness if it blew in the wrong times. Therefore it was important to do things at the proper time and in the proper season, each of which embodies its own characteristic *qi.* In the case of *wenbing*, winter is expected to be cold but if the body suffered from an internal imbalance, or if the weather is exceptionally cold, it would provide an opportunity for outside influences, in this case coldness, to enter the body and express as illness later in the spring.

For the second explanation, *Suwen* 31 stated "the *rebing* (hot diseases) nowadays are [included] within the category of *shanghan*"[9] and it was stated that they were caused by cold factors and the patient will die if the cold factor entered the *zang* and *fu*. *Nanjing* (Canon of Difficult Questions), the medical text compiled around the first or second century A.D. that actively applied the five phase theory to diseases, continued to place *wenbing* within the five categories of *shanghan* and proposed the view that the *qi* would be affected and become ill prior to the "*xue*." Both the *Huangdi neijing suwen* and *Nanjing* thus distinguished the causes and symptoms of *wenbing*, but offered only broad guidelines with a focus on movement of *qi* and *xue* within the body with acupuncture. There were no specific recommendations for pharmaceutical formulae to treat the illness.

The third explanation of *wenbing* as epidemic disorder is found in *Suwen* 71 "*liu yuan zhen ji da lun*" (Discourse on the Six Cosmic Influences) where the first development in the *taiyang* years, an unseasonal movement of the *diqi* (earthly *qi*) caused a warming trend and early growth of grasses, leading to "people becoming ill with epidemic diseases, therefore *wenbing* erupts."[10] The outbreak of *wenbing* brought about heat in the body, headaches, vomiting, eruption of boils and ulcers on the skin.[11] The cause of epidemic outbreaks was therefore connected to cosmic abnormalities rather than internal weakness of the body.

These three explanations for *wenbing* in the *Huangdi neijing* reflected the diverse traditions incorporated into the text as it was compiled over the centuries. Contradictions inevitably appeared. The notion of incubating febrile disease that manifested itself after a season seemed hard to reconcile with the notion of epidemic disorders that erupted immediately due to irregular cosmic patterns. This contradiction was not reconciled until the Qing dynasty as the *wenbing* school matured.

The *wenbing* school thus can trace its lineage to the orthodox textual tradition in medicine, but its emergence and development as an independent school of medical thought and practice owed much to *Shanghanlun* and its framework of organizing symptoms and therapy. The presentation of specific formulae for the treatment of diseases, including that of *wenbing*, emerged with the *Shanghanlun* (Treatise on Cold Damage Disorders) by Zhang Zhongjing in the early part of the third century A.D. In the preface Zhang referred to experiences with epidemic diseases where more than two hundred of his clan perished, most from cold damage illnesses. This undoubtedly influenced his perception of diseases and treatments. The *Shanghanlun* provided for the first time provided a more unified discourse on theory and practice, as well as a systematic organization of pharmaceutical formulae.

In the *Shanghanlun*, it was stated that the symptoms of *wenbing* were fever and thirst and not fearing coldness. Similar to the *Nanjing*, it distinguished the difference between the cold factor disorders and warm factor disorders, the latter being placed within the category of the *shanghan*. In treatment, the *Shanghanlun* was mainly concerned with treating the cold factor disorders though many of its treatments such as the *qingre* and *gongxia* directly affected the theories of treatment in later *wenbing* schools.

It was Wang Shuhe of the Jin who, in his reorganization and editing of the *Shanghanlun,* elaborated on the warm factor disorders and expanded the scope of *wenbing* by subdividing the categories of the disease to include the *dongwen*, *wennue*, *fengwen*, *wendu*, and *wenyi*. In addition, he also emphasized the effects of unseasonable weather upon the onset of diseases, and elaborated upon unseasonable influences on health, such as intense cold during normally warm spring, intense coolness during normally warm summers, intense heat during normally cool autumn, and intense warmth during normally cold winters. This also paved the way for more discussion concerning the impact of epidemic diseases in relation to the incubating nature of diseases.

The elaboration of *wenbing* and *shanghan* theories continued in the Han (202 B.C.–220 A.D.) and Tang (618–907) periods with important physicians such as Sun Simiao (581–682) and Wang Bing (Tang physician, exact dates unknown). Sun Simiao in his *Beiji qianjin yaofang* (Essential Formulae Worth A Thousand for Emergencies) referred to *zhangli* (pestilential epidemic) in the atmosphere as cause for illnesses and thus emphasized the importance of preventing *zhangli* from entering into the body. Although it is unclear whether this paved the way for the acceptance of later Wu Youxing's idea of *liqi* (epidemic *qi*), an external element that entered the body. One of the main themes in the works of Sun is that of prevention of illness through maintaining the *zhenqi* within the body. Bodily *xu* (emptiness) opened the way for a breakdown of health.[12] Sun and others formulated new therapies based on the notions of the outside causation of *wenrebing*. Sun advocated the use of cooling medicine to rid the body of heat (*qingre*) and to facilitate the release of poison (*jiedu*), and at the same time emphasizing the importance of nourishing the *yin* within the body to strengthen it. Therefore in protecting the vital essence within the body, one can prevent external noxious influences from entering. Both of these therapies ultimately became the basis for the treatment of *wenbing*.

The second major phase of the development of *wenbing* theory occurred in the Song (960–1279), Jin (1115–1234), and Yuan (1264–1368) periods. This coincided with an overall flourishing of medicine and the formation of major schools. Thus the *Siku quanshu zongmu tiyao* (An Abstract on the Index to the Complete Encyclopedia of the Four Divisions) commented that the various schools of medicine began in the Jin and Yuan periods when there emerged the four major theorists — the so-called Jin Yuan s*idajia* (The Four Major Schools of the Jin Yuan Period): Liu Wansu (1120?–1200), Zhang Congzheng (1156–1228), Li Gao (1180–1251), and Zhu Zhenheng (1281–1358).[13] One of the major impact on the development of these schools was the increasingly importance of the work *Shanghanlun*. The work was not widely known or accessible previously, and even Sun Simiao lamented his late acquaintance with the work. The Song government's compilation and editing of medical texts brought it out of obscurity, paving the way for the formation of the *shanghan* school. This stimulated dynamic investigations into theory and therapy.

The transmission of medical texts had suffered in the political turmoil and many were lost during upheavals in society. The Song government, due to its interest in medicine and aided in the spread of printing, undertook to print many works which had originally been lost. Much of the work was undertaken in the Imperial Medical Academy where physicians and scholars had access to a wide array of classical texts. The proliferation of medical texts paved the way and provided material for the flourishing of medical theories in the following Jin and Yuan periods. The Jin and Yuan medical theories were also stimulated by the unrest and widespread outbreak of epidemic diseases at the time. The inadequacies of existing theories provided the opportunity for the development of new ones.

Prior to the Song, different formulae were used for the treatment of cold factor and warm factor disorders, and the two diseases were often discussed separately even though the latter was often placed under the former. For example in Sun Simiao's *Beiji qianjin yaofang* (Essential Prescriptions Worth A Thousand for Emergencies) he listed over twenty formulae for the treatment of warm factor diseases which remained the basis for many later *wenbing* physicians. However in the Song with the editing of the *Shanghanlun* by Lin Yi and Gao Baoheng, many physicians used methods for treating the cold factors to treat warm factor disorders, igniting a controversy between the warm factor and cold factor schools.

Major developments in medical theory occurred both in the north and south. The northern schools were represented by the *Hejian xuepai* (School of Hejian) and the *Yishui xuepai* (School of Yishui). The *Hejian xuepai* was represented by Liu Wansu who emphasized the theory of *wuyun liuqi* (five revolving phases and six *qi)* in the *Neijing* as a comprehensive explanation for all illnesses. The five revolving phases in connection to the five *zang* determined the origins of illnesses, and the six *qi* are their manifestations.[14] This originated from his contention that *liuqi* (six *qi*) were all from *huohua* (heat transformation), thus to drive out the heat, cooling medicines were the most appropriate. He opposed the prevailing trend in using *wenzao* (warm and irritating) medicine. Liu's main contribution to the *wenbing* school therefore was in establishing the importance of *huore* within the body and the use of cooling therapies. Liu and his disciple Zhang Zhongzhen both emphasized external heat influences on the body. Liu was thus considered an important figure in the formation of the *wenbing* school.[15]

Liu's disciple Ma Zongsu passed his learning on to Zhu Zhenheng and thus transmitted the teachings of this school to the south. Ma based his theory on the *Neijing* which stated that when in the winter the body is invaded by cold, in the spring it will become *wen* illness. He based his arguments on this *Suwen* text to propound that there were no cold factor diseases, only warm factor diseases. He considered that all diseases which exhibited symptoms of fever, regardless of whether they were induced exogenously or internally, or what season it was, all would be classified as *rebing*. Therefore in the *Suwen* there were chapters on heat factors ("*relunpian*," "*cirepian*," and "*pingrebinglunpian* ") and none specifically on *shanghan*. It was emphasized that warm factor disorders had to be cured by methods for warm factor illnesses, namely, cooling therapy, and disputed the use of warming treatments. This school of thought also recognized that many of the *rebing* were contagious.

Zhu Zhenheng however emphasized more the internal development of heat, and promoted the nourishment of the *yin* essence to prevent its depletion. The *Yishui xuepai* is represented by Zhang Yuansu[16] who, although he also based his theory upon the *wuyun liuqi*, did not advocate warming factors as an illness. The southern schools were represented by the *Shanghan xuepai* (School of Cold Damage Disorders) and the *Wenre xuepai* (School of Warm/Heat Factor Disorders).

Philosophical ideas such as those of Song philosopher Zhang Zai also helped to shape the discourse on *wenbing*. He placed emphasis upon the rising and falling movement and repose of the *qi* which Zhang Yuansu adopted in elaboration on the rise and fall of the aroma of drugs. The Song philosopher Shao Yong who expounded the *xiantian* and *houtian* theories also find similar references in medicine, referring for example to the *shen* (kidney) as the basis of the *xiantian* and the *pi* (spleen) as the basis of the *houtian.* The impact of philosophy was fostered also by a surge in the publication of medical texts under patronage of the government.

This second phase in the development of the *wenbing* school therefore built upon the theoretical foundations of the previous one, and elaborated upon the need for cooling medicine and nourishment of *yin*. There was also increasing call for the separation of *wenbing* from *shanghan*.

The third phase of development during the late Ming and Qing periods represented the maturation of the *wenbing* school. One of the clear indications of this development was specialized publications specifically on *wenbing* and there was a proliferation of publications in this subject. Development of the *wenbing* school in the late Ming and Qing was heavily influenced not only by continuing discourse on causes, symptoms, and therapy, but also by intense intellectual debates over the text *Shanghanlun*. This contributed to a visible and sometimes contentious debate over whether *wenbing* was a sub-category of *shanghan*

We will begin by examining the main developments that separated *wenbing* into an independent school through the writings of physicians Yu Chang, Ye Gui, Wu Gutong, and Xue Xue. Yu Chang was especially important in establishing the three pillars of diagnosis, pointing out that there were three scenarios in which *wenbing* could occur: injured in the winter and becoming ill in the spring; not storing [one's] essence in the winter will ensure illness in the spring; and a combination of injury and not storing essence in the winter leading to a simultaneous eruption of illness in the spring.[17]

Ye Gui was probably the most famous of the four. A Suzhou physician, Ye provided the theoretical formulation of the different stages of *wenbing*: noxious influences reaching *wei, qi, ying, xue* (defensive, *qi,* constructive, *xue*) stages, each stage exhibiting different manifestations and thus requiring different approaches to therapy. In addition, Ye also contributed to more sophisticated methods of diagnosis in examination of tongue, teeth, and skin spots.

Increasing sophistication in distinguishing between *shanghan* and *wenbing* led to better diagnosis and therapy. But the separation of *wenbing* from *shanghan* also benefited from intellectual debates over *Shanghanlun* and questions over the authenticity of the work. This debate engaged physicians and scholars alike, and was instrumental in fostering an atmosphere where the establishment of an independent school was possible. In the following we will examine this issue over *Shanghanlun*.

Many recent scholars in the People's Republic categorize two main currents of thought in medicine during the Qing period: the so-called *fugu pai* (Return to Antiquity Faction)[18] and the *gexin pai* (Innovative Faction).[19] The former advocated the use of the methods of evidential learning to decipher classical medical texts, while the latter emphasized the separation of the *wenre* illness and the *shanghan* illnesses and use of cooling therapy for the former. This represented the maturation of the *wenbing* school as it breaks out of the *shanghan* framework. These labels however are the invention of scholars and there is no indication in the writings of the physicians at the time that they considered themselves adversaries of each other or consciousness of any divisions into camps.

The late Ming and the Qing periods witnessed the rise of evidential learning. During that time many scholars placed the blame for the demise of the Ming government on the Song-Ming *lixue* (Study of Moral Principles), criticizing it as overly concerned with the cultivation of self and neglecting the practical aspects of learning. In their view, there was also too much Buddhist influence in the *lixue* of the Ming which diverted much attention away from the practical affairs. There was a reaction against the Lu-Wang school of neo-Confucianism which in the view of late Ming and Qing scholars, had lost the practical aspects of the original Confucianism. Therefore there was a "back to the Han" movement which meant a return to the commentaries which the Han scholars had written concerning the Classics. This was because they believed that the Han scholars by virtue of living closer to the time of Confucius, and prior to the introduction of Buddhism into China, would be closer to the true meaning of Confucius. This was the Hanxue Movement in contrast to the Songxue of the neo-Confucians. The study by Elman also shows that the lower Yangzi region was a center of the evidential research scholars, particularly in the areas of Jiangsu, Zhejiang, and Anhui.[20]

The emphasis of the Hanxue scholars on the "correct" interpretation of ancient texts led them to adopt the tools of evidential learning to study the texts, and they made important contributions in textual criticism and philology. These methods of research became their way of restoring the past in its true form. Many scholars at this time were interested in and also published works on science and medicine, for example Song Yingxing, Fang Yizhi, Mei Wending, and Jiao Xun. However using the method of evidential research to study the medical classics was undertaken mostly by Confucian physicians.

Medicine was also influenced by the Hanxue scholars. They used the methods of the Hanxue scholars to study the *Lingshu* (Divine Pivot) and *suwen* (Basic Questions) books of the *Huangdi neijing* (Inner Canon of the Yellow Emperor) and also investigated the true meaning of the *shanghan* theory. They undertook to edit the original texts and examine the original meaning of the works. Therefore this period saw a proliferation of works which were concerned with classical medical texts such as the *Lingshu*,

Suwen, *Shanghanlun*, *Jinkui yaolue* (Essentials of the Golden Casket), and the *Shennong bencaojing* (Canon of the Divine Husbandman's Materia Medica). There was a proliferation of the annotation of these medical classics. In the Ming there were altogether fifty-nine works, and in the Qing it increased to two hundred and eighty-nine.[21] The Confucian physicians who were representative of this trend were Yu Jiayan, Zhang Jingan, Gao Shizong, Ke Yunbo, Xu Lingtai, Huang Yuanyu, and Chen Xiuyuan. In the next section we will turn our attention to the discussion on the authenticity of the *Shanghanlun.*

One common thread of the so-called *fugu pai* was that they still mainly adhered to the theories set out in the *Shanghanlun* and further elaborated upon it. Thus Ren Yingqiu still placed them under the category of the *shanghan xuepai* (School of Cold Damage Disorders). It was also due to the predominance of interest in the *Shanghanlun* which set the stage for the maturation of the *wenre* theory and in emphasis on the differences between the *shanghan* (cold damage) and *wenre* (heat damage) types of illnesses and forms of treatment.

The physicians who were prominent were Ye Tianshi, Xie Shenbai, Wu Tang, and Wang Shixiong. There will be more detailed discussion on the physicians of the *wenre* school in the later section of this chapter but here it is interesting to note that there is a difference in the background of the physicians in the *shanghan* and *wenre* schools during this period. The prominent physicians who were proponents of the *wenre* school, with the exception of Xue Shenbai, did not participate in the examinations. Xue sat for the *boxue hongci* (Erudite Literatus)[22] examination twice during the Qianlong reign (1736–1795) but did not pass.[23] He was well versed in the classics as well as good in painting. Both Ye Tianshi and Wang Shixiong came from families that had produced physicians for several generations. Therefore they could be considered as hereditary physicians in contrast to the Confucian physicians, of which many of the physicians engaged in the debate on the *Shanghanlun* could be categorized.

To cite a few examples, Xu Lingtai[24] came from a well-established family from Jiangsu and was a *zhusheng* (student) but he looked down upon the works taught and the strict writing style, and therefore he left and studied the philosophy of the *Yijing* (Book of Changes) and works of Laozi. He was skilled in fields such as astronomy and geography but especially in medicine. In 1759 he was summoned to the capital to attend to the Grand Secretary Jiang Pu and later was appointed to the Imperial Academy of Medicine (*taiyiyuan*) but returned home shortly. Yu Chang believed that Wang Shuhe's re-editing of the *Shanghanlun* did not represent the original and wrote

Shanghan shanglunpian. He was a *fubang gongsheng* (Tribute student on the Supplementary List)[25] who also disdained pursuing an official career and became a monk instead. He was famous for his skills as a physician. Huang Yuanyu was also a *zhusheng* but later turned to the study of medicine out of his anger that a quack physician had ruined his eyes. Chen Xiuyuan who defended Wang Shuhe's *Shanghanlun* as close to the original, became a *juren* (Provincial Graduate) in 1792. Ke Yunbo who wrote the *Shanghan laisuji* also was well versed in the classics and talented in poetry. He gave up being a Provincial graduate and devoted himself to the study of medicine.

Therefore it seems that during the late Ming and early Qing periods, the trend towards evidential research among scholars also deeply affected the Confucian physicians. They adopted the methodology of the School of Han Learning to study the classical medical texts. Debates among these Confucian physicians also paralleled those of the evidential scholars at the time who attempted to search for meaning at the original source. The Han Learning scholars turned to the study of classical interpretations which were closer to the Han dynasty in the belief that since they were closer to the time of the compilation of the Classics, they would be more likely to reveal the truth. The Song sources were rejected by them because they were more removed from the time when the Classics were composed. Encouraged by the Qing state, evidential research thus became "in vogue."

Confucian physicians came under the influence as well and undertook to study the ancient classical medical texts in an effort to search for the true meaning of the writings. It is perhaps therefore not surprising that most of the physicians who were engaged in evidential research in medical classics were brought up in the tradition of the *shidafu* and were expected to participate in examinations and pursue the normal route towards success. It is also not surprising that most of these Confucian physicians had rejected the normal path and undertook the study of medicine. Medicine had always been very much part of the education of a Confucian scholar, and this pursuit enabled them to participate within the dominant intellectual trends even when they did not pursue a political career. This is also in line with the tradition of Confucian scholars to engage in textual studies of medical texts. For example the Song scholars such as Zhang Zai, Su Shi, Shen Kuo, and Zhu Xi were all interested in medicine and engaged in textual editing and commentaries. Robert Hymes in his study on physicians in the Song and Yuan periods shows that medical knowledge was ratified, but it was primarily a knowledge of texts which was considered appropriate.[26]

It was mainly the hereditary physicians who were attempting to break out of the theoretical framework of the *Shanghanlun*, and they were labeled as the *gexin pai* by some medical historians.[27] However as has been mentioned above this distinction is not used by other medical historians. These physicians attempted to bring to the forefront the importance of the *wenbing* and their widespread experience undoubtedly aided in the accumulation of practical experience and knowledge which provided the basis for the development of their theories. The theory of the *wenbing* school not only developed within the dynamics of the classical medical tradition but also was related to the larger society in intellectual, social and economic trends. The impact of classical scholarship on medicine can best be illustrated by the efforts to examine the authenticity of the *Shanghanlun.*

The work of which most of the controversy was centered around among the scholars and physicians was the *Shanghanlun* (Treatise on Cold Damage disorders). This work was originally part of the *Shanghan zabinglun* (Treatise on Cold Damage and Miscellaneous Disorders) which was attributed to Zhang Ji and possibly written sometime between 196–220 A.D. It was lost in the disruption which prevailed at the end of the Han dynasty in the third century A.D. and it was later put together again during the Jin by Wang Shuhe probably some fifty or sixty years later. It was again re-edited in the tenth century and again in the eleventh century by Lin Yi. The controversy which drew sharp debates from the Confucian physicians was whether Wang Shuhe's editing of the work was true to the original or not. There were essentially two factions: those who believed that Wang Shuhe had fundamentally altered the original text and that it was no longer that which was written by Zhang Ji were represented by physicians such as Wang Yuanyu, Zhang Nan, Zhang Lu; and those who believed that the Wang Shuhe version was basically true to the original, were represented by physicians such as Zhang Jingan and Chen Xiuyuan.

The reason for this renewed level of interest in a work that had remained in relative obscurity during the Sui and Tang periods can be first traced back to the Song's private and governmental efforts at editing medical works and the improvements in printing.[28] In the Song there were approximately 42 works focusing on the *Shanghanlun*, in Jin fourteen, in Yuan eleven, and in Ming it increased to fifty-one and Qing has sixty-six.[29] In the Ming and Qing the emergence of evidential research brought about an earnest debate on the authenticity of the text itself.

The controversy which drew sharp debates from the Confucian physicians was whether Wang Shuhe's editing of the work was true to the original or not. There were essentially two factions: those who believed that Wang Shuhe had fundamentally altered the original text and that it was no longer that which was written by Zhang Zhongjing. This faction is represented by physicians such as Wang Yuanyu, Zhang Nan. The other group believed that even though the Wang Shuhe version may be different from what Zhang Zhongjing had written, it was basically true to the original.

Ming physician Fang Youzhi (1523–?) lamented the corruption of Zhang Zhongjing's work by Wang Shuhe in the Jin (266–316) and then by Zheng Wuji in the Jin (1115–1234). He spent over twenty years studying the *Shanghanlun* and wrote *Shanghanlun tiaobian* (Treatise on Cold Damage Disorders: Systematic critical examination) in which he carefully reconstituted the work and systematically examined each sentence/word. It marked one of the major attempts to rediscover the *Shanghanlun* before its revision by the later Jin and Song editors. It also became the basis for which the late Ming early Qing physician Yu Chang (1585–1664) wrote his *Shanghan Shanglunpian* (A Respectful Discourse on the *Shanghanlun*), printed in 1648, a work which later became popular.[30] In the preface to the *Shanghanlun tiaobian*, Fang comments:

> Medicine became the Way starting with the Bencaojing. The Su, Nan[31] explained it clearly, and it is completed by the *Shanghanlun.*[32]

Although before Fang's work came out there had been scholars and physicians working on *Shanghanlun*, yet it was Fang who ignited the debate concerning the authenticity and validity of Wang Shuhe's edition. However there are also people who dispute the reconstitution of the work by people like Fang Youzhi and Yu Chang only served to go against the original intentions of Zhang Zhongjing. For example Ke Yunbo, in his *Shanghan laisuji* (Renewal of the treatise on Cold Damaged Disorders) commented that the book *Shanghanlun* after Wang Shuhe's rearrangement was no longer the original book written by Zhang Ji. He believes that much of the original had been lost, and that Wang had added much of his own to the work. Later interferences of the text made the originally simple theory of Zhang Ji something difficult to understand. Thus he believes that in order to properly understand the true meaning in the work, one must "concentrate one's attention and settle the mind, used wisdom to observe silently, carefully espouse each section. Investigate thoroughly each sentence, which are the words of Zhongjing, which are the writing of Shuhe, if there are missing things, inverted sentences, wrong characters, excess passages, all these should be pointed out, then it will immediately let the true face of the author appear from the words and sentences."[33] Ke Qin also pointed out that in the original preface by Zhang Ji, the *Shanghan zabinglun* had altogether sixteen *juan*, thus showing that s*hanghan* and *zabing* were not separated into two books. The items which were not labeled as *shanghan* would then be under the category of *zabing*.

Other physicians, however, do not cater to the view that Wang Shuhe had corrupted the original. Xu Dachun believes that the original has already been lost and Wang Shuhe's rearrangement is reliable. He accuses those people who want to change and making things more obscure in the process instead.[34] Chen Xiuyuan (1766–1833) also thinks that Wang Shuhe made a major contribution in his editing of the *Shanghanlun*, and even though he added in works of his won, his intention was to supplement the original text to make it more detailed and did not intend to mislead people.

Therefore it seems that during the late Ming and Qing periods, the trend towards evidential research among scholars also deeply affected the physicians as well. They adopted the methodology of the School of Han Learning to study the classical medical texts. Debates among these physicians also paralleled those of the evidential scholars at the time who attempted to search for meanings at the original source. The Han Learning scholars turned to the study of classical interpretations which were closer to the Han dynasty in the belief that since they were closer to the time of the compilation of the Classics, they would be more likely to reveal the truth. The Song sources were rejected by them because they were more removed from the time when the Classics were composed. Encouraged by the Qing state, evidential research thus became `in vogue' and engaged by intellectuals.

For the physicians, although Wang Shuhe's editing of *Shanghanlun* was done during the Jin (266–316), it already raised the serious question of whether it was true to the original or not. The significance of this debate is that it brought the *Shanghanlun* into the limelight. It came to be mentioned alongside the medical classics such as the *Neijing*, the *Shennong bencaojing*, and the *Nanjing*. Zhang Zhongjing himself was portrayed as the successor of the work of the sages and has been elevated to the position of a sage. His role in medicine has often been compared to that of Confucius in the Confucian tradition in that he was the one who inherited and expounded upon the medical tradition of the Yellow Emperor and the Divine Husbandman and in turn paved the way for later physicians. For example Fang Youzhi comments that Zhang Zhongjing has been venerated as the sage of medicine (*yisheng*).[35]

Therefore it is evident that one of the major topics of discussion among the Qing physicians revolved around the *Shanghanlun*. This not only indicates a renewed level of interest in the work itself but it also underscores the fact that within the classical medical tradition, a general sense of dissatisfaction has emerged concerning how the systems of knowledge have been classified and systematized. The early and mid-Ming has generally been characterized by a continuation of the tradition from the Song-Jin-Yuan periods, but beginning from late Ming, there was a renewed interest and reevaluation of *Shanghanlun.* Zhang Zhongjing's followers became one of the 'schools' in the medical tradition. But in Qing his view were further elevated to the level of *jing* by physicians such as Xu Dachun and his colleagues.

The attempt to elevate it to the level of a canon is perhaps also an effort to elevate the status and position of medicine in society. Theoretically, many of the developments in medicine can trace their intellectual lineage back to the Four Major Schools and ultimately to Zhang Zhongjing. Thus the elevation of Zhang Zhongjing and the portrayal of him as a sage and founding father in medicine as discussed in Chapter One, making him the Confucius of the medical tradition not only gives more credibility to their own work but also puts medicine on a par with the dominant intellectual tradition.

Wu Youxing and *Wenyi lun*

The infectious nature of the *wenbing* was given its major advancement in theory by the late Ming physician Wu Youxing[36] and represented a major breakthrough in the third stage of development of the *wenbing* school. He personally experienced the series of epidemics which ravaged the empire around 1408–1643 [37] and saw the inadequacies of treatment using the *shanghan* method. Therefore from the cases he came across he examined the causes for the diseases and put forward his argument that epidemics were not to be explained solely by reference to the year and season, and they were not caused by the invasion of the *liuyin*. But rather they were caused by *liqi* which entered the human body through the nose and mouth.

His *Wenyilun*[38] was written around 1642 and its importance and significance has been recognized by physicians and medical historians. His book investigated the contagious character of the epidemics, the causes, how they were transmitted, changes during transmission and methods of cure. He believed that *wenyi* was basically a *rebing*. He disagreed with Wang Shuhe who said that epidemics were caused by unseasonable weather: i.e., that when it was spring and should be warm but is cold instead; when it was summer and should be hot but was cool instead; when it was fall and should be cool but was hot instead; and when it was winter and should be cold but was warm instead. These he believed were natural changes in the weather and even though there may be differences, they were still within the normal range and unseasonable weather would only cause external illnesses and did not cause epidemics.

The real cause of epidemics he believed was a kind of *liqi* in the atmosphere which would invade regardless of old and young, healthy and sick. This *liqi* enters the people's bodies through the mouth and nose. This *liqi* is but one kind of the *zaqi* which is prevalent in the atmosphere. Thus seasonal changes, contrary to accepted wisdom, was not the determining factor. He comments in the essay on "*zaqilun*" that:

> But these qi have no form by which we can perceive them, still less any sound or smell. How can we see or hear them? How can man know of their existence? They come when they will and strike where they will. If the people clash against them, they produce the various diseases, each according to its nature...
>
> Generally speaking, when a disease is widespread throughout a given region so that from one household to the next and throughout whole families everyone is afflicted in the same way, this is the work of a `seasonally current epidemic qi — that is, a concentration of one of the miscellaneous *qi*...
>
> Explanation of the prevalence of diseases cannot be confined to consideration of the year and the seasons, for it is not something that can be determined by the procession of the Five Agents or the vagaries of the Six *qi*,[39] which is how we know that in their advent the *qi* are arbitrary with regard to time...[40]

Although the difference between *shanghan* and *wenyi* is quite striking, yet Wu Youxing recognized that sometimes they are difficult to distinguish from each other. If the heteropathy of the *yiqi* has invaded the stomach, then the symptoms exhibited would be somewhat similar. Therefore in his essay on "*bianming shanghan shiyi* " (distinguishing between cold factor disorders and epidemics) he pointed out that *shanghan* is always caused by being injured by cold such as dressing too thinly, being drenched by rain, undressing in the wind and so on which induced coldness and shivering and a fear of the wind and cold, pain in the body and head and fever. As for epidemic diseases there are no outside causes as above but a general feeling of faintness with fever but no fear of the cold. The *shanghan* is not contagious yet the epidemic is contagious; the *shanghan* enters the body through the skin and the epidemic diseases enters through the mouth and nose; the *shanghan* symptoms are manifested immediately, but the epidemic diseases will only be manifested after some time. In treatment, he says that for *shanghan* one can induce sweating but not for the epidemic diseases. For *shanghan* if there are the appearance of a rash then the illness is serious, but for the other, it shows a release of the disease. The major difference between *shanghan* and epidemic diseases is the different areas of the body in which the heteropathy (*xie*) is located. Due to the fact that there are differences for the transmission of the disease and also the path of the disease, the bodily constitution of the patient, there should be different ways of treatment, and Wu Youxing classified them into nine categories (*jiu chuan*) with separate treatment for each.

Therefore Wu was able to make detailed observations of epidemic diseases because of his experiences which enabled him to obtain a deeper understanding of the nature and transmission of these diseases, so that he was able to formulate a more efficient system of treatment. With his observations and influenced by the *hejian* school, he concluded that epidemic diseases were a kind of warm factor disorders and also traced this back to the *Neijing*. He also espoused that *wenyi* is the epidemic form of *wenbing* and proposed that *wenyi* and *wenre* are the same. His theory that the heteropathy entered the body from the mouth and nose paved the way for Ye Tianshi's development of the theory that the warm heteropathy first attacked the *fei* (lung) and then was transmitted to the *xinbao* (heart).

Many medical textbooks for TCM in China hail Wu Youxing as an early advocate of the germ theory and contagion, more than two hundred years ahead of Lister and Pasteur.[41] Yet is it clear from our discussion of Wu's ideas that he did not emphasize contagion, but the independence from seasonal happenings. This clearly challenged the deep-rooted belief in the importance of seasons in causing illness, as emphasized in the *Huangdi neijing*.. Wu's importance is in seeking legitimation not from the orthodox textual tradition, but rather from practical observation, and challenging the *shanghan* tradition.

A Southern Tradition

The maturation of the *wenbing* school was made possible by the theoretical developments based upon previous attempts to place it in a separate category from the *shanghan* disorders and to employ treatment appropriate to the disease. It seems that the physicians who were the chief advocates of the *wenbing* school at this time belonged to the category of hereditary physicians whereas many of those who were engaged in the debates on the *Shanghanlun* using the methods of evidential research were Confucian physicians. In her work on the *wenbing* school, Marta Hanson has emphasized the importance of an epistemological shift to local medical traditions, reflecting a rise in regional identity in the later part of the nineteenth century and a resistance against the centralizing force of the state. Thus the invention of *wenbing* as a southern tradition was important culturally as well as politically.[42] This north-south divergence and creation of separate identity was not new and can be seen in the creation of northern and southern types of foot *qi* in the thirteenth century. In her study on the changing conceptions of foot *qi*, Hilary Smith suggests that it was due to both political factors as well as metaphysical influences.[43]

The most important proponent of the *wenbing* school in the Qing was Ye Tianshi (1666–1745).[44] He came from a family of physicians and his grandfather Ye Shi was said to be the first of the family to specialize in medicine. As a youngster Ye studied the classics and in his spare time also received medical training from his father. There is no mention in any of the sources that he took any examinations and his name is not in the *Ming-Qing Jinshi timingzhuan* (Biographies of the Presented Scholars of the Ming and Qing). After his father died he received his training from one of his father's pupils by the surname of Zhu. He was said to be exceptionally brilliant and understood quickly and soon surpassed his teachers. He became a skilled physician and one of the most respected of his time.

Ye Tianshi however wrote very little and most of the works that bear his name were either compiled by his followers or falsely attributed to him. After his death his followers edited a collection of his cases and prescriptions entitled *Linzheng zhinan yian* (Collection of Medical Cases for A Guide to Diagnosis). A book entitled *Wenre lunzhi* (Treatise on Warm/Heat Factor Disorders) is also attributed to him. Ye Tishi's most important contribution to the development of the *wenbing* theory is that he proposed four stages of development of the disease: *wei*, *qi* , *ying* , *xue* , which Sivin translates as: the defensive sector, the active *qian* sector, the constructive *qi* sector, and the blood sector. The stages of development in the progression of illness are

> The special features of defensive *qi* sector disorders are fever and abnormal sensitivity to cold, headache, tongue coating thin and whitish, and pulse floating or floating and accelerated. Those of the active qi sector are strong (that is) high fever without abnormal sensitivity to cold, perspiration, dry mouth with desire to drink, red tongue with yellow coating, pulse swollen and accelerated or sunken and full. Those of the constructive *qi* sector are fever rising during the night, agitation, mind half-beclouded, raving, little thirst, in some cases a barely perceptible rash, tongue crimson with little or no coating, and pulse small and accelerated. Those of the blood sector are—on a foundation of those of the constructive sector—confused state of mind; sometimes agitation or manic behavior; clearly perceptible rash; and in serious cases vomiting of blood; blood in the stool or urine and other hemorrhagic

symptoms; tongue tissues crimson or purple and dry; coating absent; and pulse sunken, small, and accelerated.[45]

Another important figure in the development of the *wenbing* theory is Xue Shengbai who had failed the *boxue hongci* degree and devoted himself to medicine. The work *Wenre tiaobian* (Systematic Manifestation Type Determination in Warm/Heat Factor Disorders) is attributed to him although the exact authorship cannot be ascertained. There are altogether forty-six types of manifestations, the theories of which were mainly developed based upon the description of symptoms and manifestation. Xue was particularly experienced with the warm and wet type of disorders *wenshi* and distinguished between warm type disorders and wet types.

Wu Tang (1736–1820), one of the prominent physicians experienced in warm factor disorders personally witnessed several infectious febrile illnesses in the area, and this prompted him to devote himself to study the warm factor disorders. He compiled the *Wenbing tiaobian.* He believed that the difference between *shanghan* and *wenbing* was a difference between fire and water. The former type of disorders originated in water whereas the latter originated in fire. Therefore because the heteropathy responsible for warm factor disorders was caused by fire and entered the body through the mouth and nose, thus it was the *fei* (gold) which was first affected and thus it was fire against gold. Therefore diagnosis and treatment should not follow that of Zhang Ji's *Shanghanlun* but should use Liu Hejian's *sanjiao fenzhengfa.* It was also important to use bitter and cooling therapy for treatment since the disorder damages the yin of the body.

Wang Shixiong (1808–1890) was a later contemporary among the Qing physicians and also came from a family of physicians. He was noted for his work on *huoluan* which ravaged the country from the 1820s onward. He distinguished between epidemic *huoluan* and non-epidemic *huoluan.* The causes of epidemic *huoluan* he believed was due to a kind of heteropathy which was mainly to be found in unclean water, the drinking of which would cause the illness. He particularly cited the example of Shanghai which was crowded and filthy from the accumulation of dirt in nearby rivers and water sources, thus contributing to the spread of *huoluan* in the city. Since the disease often occurred during the hot summer months of the year and the environment was crowded and humid, once the diseases started it spread quickly to other places. From the symptoms he concluded that most of the cases belonged to the *shire* category, and because of this it often resulted in cramps. This type of *huoluan* was the *re* type, to be distinguished from the *han* type.

The physicians of the *wenbing* school were concerned with the separation of the warm type of disorder from the cold type based chiefly upon their observation of symptoms in illnesses. Treatments and remedies were used to restore the balance of the body which had been disturbed by the disorder. Incorrect diagnosis of the disorder and the use of the *shanghan* method of treatment was very dangerous for the patient. Thus the *wenbing* physicians used the accumulated knowledge and experience from their treatment of patients to formulate a new type of diagnosis and treatment. Their concepts and theories were still very much based upon the theoretical framework set down in the *Neijing*. Although most Qing physicians would not dispute the existence of the *han* type of disorders, the significance of their theories lay in the fact that they brought out the importance of the warm factor disorders and extracted it from the *shanghan* tradition to establish it as an independent school of thought in its own right.

It has been discussed that medieval economic revolution brought about an emergence of intellectual activity which was centered particularly in the Jiangnan region. Similarly in medicine, the shift of economic, political and intellectual activity to the south beginning in the mid-Tang, there was a gradual emergence of the prominence of physicians from the south.

As will be discussed later, the late Ming and Qing witnessed a surge in the number of physicians in the Suzhou area. The concentration of physicians has roughly parallel the development of urban centers in the region, in particular Suzhou, though situated in the southern region, have been the center of economic development for a long period of time and this perhaps also accounts for the predominance of physicians from this area. Both Ye Tianshi and Xue Shengbai came from Wuxian. Most of the physicians in this area were either Confucian physicians or hereditary physicians.

The elite medical tradition in China was based very much in its texts and the development of medical theories was brought about both by the evolution in the internal dynamics of the theoretical framework itself, aided by the accumulation of knowledge and experience, and by interaction and mutual influence with the larger society in the intellectual, social and economic fields. The gradual accumulation of medical experience and the epidemics which were widespread in the late Ming periods helped to stimulate the physicians to seek alternative diagnosis and treatment. Many of the physicians advocating the *wenbing* theory themselves personally witnessed several large scale epidemics. For example Wu Youxing, Wu Tang, and Wang Shixiong all were able to make use of their experience to further substantiate and legitimate the *wenbing* theory which had been systematically propounded beginning in the Jin and Yuan periods through the experience gained in their practices.

The intellectual trends at the time which placed much emphasis upon the study of the *Shanghanlun* also helped to stimulate their interest in formulating the theory. The Confucian physicians, although they disdained participation in the examinations and a normal route to success, nevertheless kept themselves within the dominant intellectual current through their study of the *Shanghanlun* using the methodology of evidential research. It was mostly the hereditary physicians who were able to break away from the confines of traditional theory and unburdened by a need to participate in the dominant intellectual activities of the society.

The emergence of the *wenbing* school also reflected the shift of intellectual, social and economic activities from the north to the south, beginning in the mid-Tang period. It represented a major challenge to the hitherto dominant southern tradition of the *shanghan* school. This rise in the importance of especially the Jiangnan region can be seen in the surge in the number of physicians in this area during the Ming and Qing periods. There is much that still could be done in looking into the relationship between the economical and social developments of this region with the development of medicine in this area, and perhaps the role region played in formulating the theoretical advancements. It has traditionally been held that south China was more prone to outbreaks of epidemic diseases and there have been studies on the widespread worship of plague gods of this area which reflected the prevalence of epidemics.[46]

The emergence of the *wenbing* school as a separate school of thought in the Ming and Qing therefore reflected the complex interplay between theory and practice, and the fluid boundaries among the different groups of physicians. Even though the Confucian physicians wanted to elevate themselves above all other medical practitioners, they nevertheless engaged intellectually and at a practical level with other groups of physicians, most notably the hereditary physicians.

The medical landscape in late imperial China reflected the increased competition in medical practice in the Jiangnan region and anxiety on part of those who considered themselves *ruyi* (Confucian physicians). This led to debates over the qualifications of the ideal physician and the effort to construct a medical lineage with Zhang Zhongjing as the medical sage (Chapter One). Even though the late imperial state in China did not establish licensing laws for the practice of medicine, their interest and patronage of medicine is reflected in the construction of the *sanhuang miao* (Temple of the Three Emperors) and in state sponsorship of the publication of medical texts (Chapter Two). But even as the state endorsed the orthodox medical lineage that is traced to the Three Emperors, the development of medical practice, theory, and therapy were shaped by close interaction with local beliefs and experiences provided for another source of legitimation.

Notes

[1] This inclusion of epidemic diseases and their symptoms within the *wenbing* category was not unchallenged. Lei Feng in his *Shibing lun* (A Discussion on Epidemic Diseases) emphasized the differences between *wen* (heat factor) and *wen* (epidemic), see his "Wen wen bu tong lun." (A Discussion on the difference between *wen* and *wen*). Wang Dexuan argued that it was Wu Youxing and the publication of his work *Wenyilun* that contributed to a confusion between *wenbing* and *wenyi*, the latter having very different causes and methods of cure from the former. See Wang Dexuan, *Wenbing zhengzong* (The Orthodox Tradition of *Wenbing*), edited based on 1936 edition (Beijing: Zhongyi guji chubanshe, 1987), pp. 18–20,

[2] Hanson, *Inventing a Tradition in Chinese Medicine.*

[3] Mann, *The Talented Women of the Zhang Family*, pp. 37–38.

[4] This work was compiled over a century or more and put together in the first century B.C. or early first century A.D. It is mainly a tradition representing the Yellow River region and it uses the *yinyang* dichotomy quite extensively. The *Hanshu* (History of Han) by Ban Gu (32–92 A.D.) listed seven canonical works on medicine but among them, the only one which is extant today is the *Huangdi neijing.* There have been references to a *Waijing* (Outer Canon) and other books also but what is extant today is the *Suwen* (Basic Questions) and the *Lingshu* (Divine Pivot). Although some authors have raised doubts as to whether the extant *Lingshu* and *Suwen* were the original Canon of the Yellow Emperor. See Wu Kaopan, "Huangdi neijing, suwen, lingshu kao" (A Study of the Canon of the Yellow Emperor, Suwen and Lingshu) in *Zhonggua yishi zazhi*, 13.2: 85–87.

The development of the various writings and different theories were mostly based upon these two works. This embodied the accumulation of the different theories which existed in the *Chunqiu zhanguo* (Spring and Autumn and Warring States) period. It shows that the development of medicine by the end of this period was already emerging from practical experiences to attempt to formulate a systematic way of classifying and codifying the accumulated knowledge. The *Huangdi neijing* was the epitome of these first attempts and became the basis for the development of more sophisticated medical theories. Writers and physicians have not only produced extensive works on editing and annotating these classics in medicine, but the development of medical theories especially after the Jin and Yuan periods all traced their roots to the *Neijing.*

[5] *Huangdi neijing suwen jichu* (Collected Annotation of the *Huangdi neijing suwen*) in *Zhongguo yixue dacheng* (A Comprehensive Collection of Chinese Medical Works) ed. by Cao Bingchang (Changsha: Yuelu shushe, 1990 first printing), vol. 1, p. 145.

[6] *Suwen 3*, translation from Veith, p. 108.

[7] Ibid. See Kuriyama, "The Imagination of Winds and the Development of the Chinese Conception of the Body," in Angela Zito and Tani Barlow eds. *Body, Subject and Power in China* (Chicago: University of Chicago Press, 19940, pp. 34–38.

[8]Unschuld, 2003, pp. 183–198.

[9] *Huangdi neijing suwen jichu* 31, p. 185.

[10] *Huangdi neijing suwen jichu* 71, p. 261.

[11] Ibid.

[12] Sun Simiao, *Qianjin yifang, juan* 15.

[13] *Siqu quanshu congmu tiyao*, vol.2 (Shanghai: The Commercial Press, 1955), p. 85.

[14] Liu Wansu, *Suwen xuanji yuanbing shi* , 1186 in *Jin Yuan sidajia yixue quanshu* vol.1 (Tianjin: Tianjin kexue jishu chubanshe, 1999).

[15] For a discussion on the mechanisms of transmission of Liu's teachings from the twelfth to the fifteen centuries, see Wu Yiyi, "A Medical Line of Many Masters: A Prosopographical Study of Liu Wansu and His Disciples from the Jin to the Early Ming" in *Chinese Science* 11 (1993–94): 36–65.

[16] Date unknown, contemporary of Liu Wansu but perhaps a little later.

[17] Yu Chang, *Shanglun pian*,

[18] These labels were probably coined by later scholars and historians and I have been unable as yet to find any mention of these factions in the writings of contemporary physicians. Ren Yingqiu in his work *Zhongyi gejia xueshuo* simply does not use this term and classifies those of the *fugu* faction under the *shanghan* school, and *gexin* faction under the *wenre* school.

[19]In this book I have not dealt with the impact of western medicine on traditional Chinese medicine and its influence upon the development of medical theories principally because there has been little evidence of influence of western medicine on the development of the *wenbing* theory. The appearance of cholera, which first appeared in China in the 1820s, did play a major part in the Qing *wenbing* advocate Wang Shixiong's writings.

[20] Benjamin A. Elman, *From Philosophy to Philology—Intellectual and Social Aspects of Change in Late Imperial China* (Cambridge: Council on east Asian Studies, Harvard University, 1984), p. 6. See also Kai-wing Chow, "Purist Hermeneutics and Ritualist Ethics in Mid-Ch'ing Thought" in *Cosmology, Ontology, and Human Efficacy: Essays in Chinese Thought*, ed. by Richard J. Smith and D.W.K. Kwok (Honolulu: University of Hawaii Press, 1993): 179–204, for a discussion on anti-heterodoxy and ritualism eighteenth-century China.

[21]This figure is taken from Li Jingwei and Li Zhidong, *Zhongguo gudai yixue shilue* (A Brief History of Ancient Medicine in China), (Hebei: Kexue Jishu Chubanshe, 1990), p. 341. Their figure was calculated from the works collected in *Quanguo zhongyishu lianhe mulu* (Combined Catalogue of Works on Chinese Medicine Throughout the Country).

[22] This special degree was formally established during the *shaoxing* reign (Song Gaozong 1131–1162). The attainment of this degree required a broad range of knowledge and had produced many learned scholars.

[23] *Ershiliushi yijia zhuanji xinzhu* (New Annotation of the Biographies of Physicians in the Twenty-six Histories) (Shenyang: Liaoning University Press, 1986), p. 302.

[24] *Ershiliushi yijiacChuanji xinzhu*, pp.306–309.

[25] According to Charles O. Hucker, *A dictionary of Official Titles in Imperial China* (Stanford: Stanford University Press, 1985), pp. 294–295. A tribute student was a student under the Directorate of Education (*Guozijian*) nominated by local Confucian schools. Although they faced increasing competition from examination candidates in obtaining a good official career, they remained one of those considered "Regular Paths." A supplementary list in the Ming was a rare bulletin which was published alongside lists of men who had

passed the provincial examination to announce the extraordinary conferment of the *jinshi* degree (Metropolitan Graduate) on an outstanding passer. (Hucker, p. 219)

[26] Robert Hymes, "Not Quite Gentlemen? Doctors in Sung and Yuan" in *Chinese Science*, 8 (1987): 9–76.

[27] For example Du Congming in his *Zhongxi yixue shilue* (A Short History of Chinese and Western Medicine) (Taibei: Zhonghua dadian pianinhui, 1966) labels Chen Xiuyuan, Huang Yuanyu, Ke Yunbo, and Yu Jiayan as the *fugu pai* and Ye Tianshi, Wu Tang, Wang Shixiong as the *gexin pai.* The *Zhongguo yixueshi* (Taibei: Yuantong tushu gongshi, 1956) labels them *gupai* (Ancient Faction) and *jinpai* (Modern Faction).

[28] The Song government was an active force in the dissemination of medical knowledge and marked the height of governmental interest in health care for the people. In an attempt to organize the enormous accumulation of prescriptions, the Song government's edification and publication of the *Taiping huimin hejijufang* (Prescriptions of the Taiping Benevolent Dispensary) provided over seven hundred prescriptions for over fourteen categories of diseases and illnesses. It became very popular and was widely utilized by physicians. However it also provoked a reaction against the use of formulae for illnesses without taking into account the patient's heating, cooling, body constitution, or the state of depletion or repletion of the body's vital resources. It did not provide for a satisfactory basis for diagnosis. The so-called Jin-Yuan schools that emerged later were often reactions against the use of the *jufang*. For example Liu Wansu (1110/20?–1200) and also of Zhu Zhenheng (1281–1358).

[29] Chen Lifu, *Zhonghua Yiyao xueshi* (The Medical History of China) (Taibei: Shangwuin shuguan, 1982), p. 69.

[30] *Siqu Quanshu Congmu tiyao*, v. 2, pp. 19–20.

[31] Referring to the *Suwen* and the *Nanjing*

[32] Fang Youzhi, *Shanghanlun tiaobian*, preface 1589, printed 1592, *Zhongguo yixue dacheng xupian*, p. 53.

[33] Ke Qin, *Shanghan laisuji*, preface 1729 (Shanghai: Kexue jishu chubanshem 1986), p. 1.

[34] Xu Dacun, *Yixue yuanliulun*, p. 9b.

[35] Fang Youzhi, *Shanghanlun tiaobian*, preface.

[36] Wu Youxing, *zi* Youke. He was a native of Zhenze. A county in the present day province of Jiangsu.

[37] According to the *Mingshi* from around 1408–1643 a series of epidemics ravaged the empire. In about 1642 the epidemics hit areas of Shantong, Zhejiang, northern and southern Zhili. According to local gazetteers the Jiangnan areas also were repeatedly affected by epidemic and it had been said that several hundred families perished and sometimes whole families succumbed to the epidemic diseases. Helen Dunstan in her article "The Late Ming Epidemics: A Preliminary Survey" provides some detailed discussion on especially the epidemics in the 1580s and 1640s. An article by Imura Kôzen, "Chihôshi ni kisaiseraretaru Chûgodu ekirei ryakkô" in the *Chûgai iji shimpô* gives a relatively detailed chronology of epidemics which had occurred in China based chiefly on information contained in the local gazetteers.

[38] Nathan Sivin translates it as *Treatise on Warm-factor Epidemic Disorders (Traditional Medicine in Contemporary China*, Ann Arbor: Center for Chinese Studies, University of Michigan, 1987: p. 151). Wu Lien-teh and Wong K. Chi-min translates it as *On Plague* (*History of Chinese Medicine*, 2nd edition, Shanghai: National Quarantine Service, 1936: p. 128).

[39] This is Dunstan's translation of *wuyun liuqi.*

[40] This translation is taken from Helen Dunstan "The Late Ming Epidemics."

[41] For example, *Zhongyi gejia xueshuo* (Teachings of the Various Schools in Chinese Medicine) compiled by Chen Dashun (Hubei kexue jishu chubanshe, 1989), p. 236.

[42] Marta Hanson, "Robust Northerners and Delicate Southerners: The Nineteenth-Century Invention of a Southern Medical Tradition" in *Positions* volume 6 no. 3 (Winter 1998): 515–550.

[43] Hilary Smith, *Foot Qi: History of a Chinese Medical Disorder* (PhD Dissertation, University of Pennsylvania, 2008), pp. 142–160.

[44] Ye Gui was a native of Wuxian in Jiangsu province, however his ancestors were originally from Xi *xian* (in present day Anhui province). None of the sources, though, give an indication of when his ancestors moved to Jiangsu.

[45] Translated by Nathan Sivin, *Traditional Medicine in Contemporary China,* pp. 380–381.

[46] For example Paul Katz has studied the development of the cult of Marshal Wen in Zhejiang in relation to epidemics. Paul R. Katz, *Demon Hordes and Burning Boats: The Cult of Marshal Wen in Late Imperial Chekiang* (New York: State University of New York Press, 1995).

PART TWO

Medicine in Late Imperial Suzhou

CHAPTER FOUR

Suzhou Physicians

Proverb:

Above there is heaven,
On earth there is Suzhou and Hangzhou.

WHEN Suzhou native, Song politician, and scholar, Fan Zhongyan, claimed becoming a physician as an acceptable alternative to an official career, he probably did not foresee the number of scholars who would pursue the path to becoming physicians in the late Ming and Qing dynasties. Medical treatises written during this time almost invariably quoted Fan's motto in their prefaces. It is a curious declaration of the sentiment of an unfulfilled ambition yet also an assertion of the importance of medicine and its acceptability as replacement for an official career. Its ubiquitous use reflects the continued attempt to accord medicine with the same kind of prestige as that of an official career. The physicians' strategies to legitimize their positions versus other kinds of healers is closely tied to their shared intellectual and social heritage with the scholar officials. The effort to enhance their social status by claiming the label *ruyi* (Confucian physicians) and legitimize their practice by claiming textual authority has been discussed in Chapter One. Here we will examine the medical landscape in Suzhou where Confucian physicians, hereditary physicians, and other types of healers actively wrote and practiced medicine.

Suzhou in late imperial China was not only the center of cultural and economic activities, it was also home to an increasing number of physicians and center of a lively medical discourse. This phenomenon was manifested in the dramatic increase in the number of physicians recorded in sources such as the local gazetteers for the Ming and Qing. Since these sources were concerned mainly with elite physicians, this should not be taken as an indication of the increase in the overall number of physicians, but evidence that more members of the elite were engaged in medical activities. This however was significant in itself because the influx of scholars into medicine changed the dynamics of discourse and fostered an emerging sense of community. As discussed in Chapter three, Suzhou physicians were at the forefront of the formation of an independent *wenbing* school.

This chapter will first examine some of the social and economic factors that led to an increase in elite participation in medicine, and secondly look at the physicians in Suzhou and their community, finally examining the emerging sense of a community of this expanding group of physicians. The publishing boom that flourished in the lower Yangzi region was instrumental not only in providing a forum for discussion among the physicians, but at the same time fostered a sense of community and identity through the written dialogue. The *Wuyi huijiang* (Collected Discourses of Suzhou Physicians) was a unique publication that provided a public forum for the various groups of physicians to share and circulate their ideas, showing that despite different backgrounds, these physicians subscribed to the broader identity of *yi*.

Suzhou in Late Imperial China

Suzhou is often referred to as Wu or Wuzhong, the name dates back to the sixth century B.C. when it was built as the capital of Wu in the Spring and Autumn period. Suzhou then underwent numerous administrative changes.[1] In the Ming it had under its jurisdiction seven counties and in the Qing it was increased to nine, attesting to expansion in the region.[2] Suzhou city itself (Wu, Changzhou, and Yuanhe counties), the site of our focus, was the epitome of growth and change. Population growth in Suzhou mirrored the national tend. An influx of immigrants and sojourners, attracted by economic opportunities, also contributed to the rapid increase, making Suzhou one of the leading urban centers in late imperial times.[3]

Late imperial Suzhou experienced tremendous economic development and changes to the demography of the city. Agriculturally, Suzhou is located within the Yangzi Rice-Wheat Region.[4] Rich soil complemented by a mild climate and adequate rainfall meant favorable farming conditions and double-cropping was practiced extensively. It was also the region which for centuries had been the main producer of rice not just for itself, but for the whole nation. This was reflected in the popular saying, "When crops in Suzhou and Huzhou[5] ripen, there will be enough for all under heaven."

The scene gradually changed however as the silk and cotton industries developed, leading to a commercialization of grain so that by the eighteenth century, the region got most of its rice through imports.[6] Sericulture was central to the economy of Suzhou and mulberry trees along the dikes were a familiar feature. Peasant families engaged actively in raising silkworms and silk weaving. Increasingly, however, much of the work was being done by hired labor. The idyllic picture of a farming community was replaced by one in which there was a growing complexity of the farm economy and a resultant shift towards a more heterogeneous society in late imperial Jiangnan. Multi-layered land ownership was common in the region and it brought about a more detached form of landlord-tenant relationship. Many landlords moved into the city of Suzhou, leaving the management of the land to a manager. Scholars have noted, "this shift paralleled and encouraged a slow trend from Ming times toward elimination of fixed statuses and increased mobility of labor and land."[7] Many gentry families chose new careers with the increasing commercialization of the economy in the region. As will be elaborated later in this chapter, one of these choices was to become a physician.

Located on the Yangzi floodplain, Suzhou's proximity to the rich resources of Lake Taihu and accessibility to the Grand Canal and other river systems placed it at an advantageous position in trade and commerce. Goods from other regions of China flowed into the area, as is apparent from the stone inscriptions on *nanbeihuo ye* (the north-south commodities trade) which reflected an active trade in commodities from different regions.[8] One of the commodities was herbal medicine.

Foreign trade also played a major role in the economy of Suzhou and large amounts of silver flowed into the region. The monetization of the economy[9] and growth of the rural marketing structure brought about a greater fluidity in terms of status within the social classes. Many gentry also actively engaged in trade and other enterprises. Some scholars have come to the view that in late imperial China, "merchants and gentry were virtually fused."[10] There were many instances of gentry and merchants forming alliances through marriage. In her study on the ledgers of merit and demerit which were popular in the sixteenth and seventeenth centuries, Cynthia Browkaw argues that "to some degree merchant status was now glorified as a positive achievement in itself, one that might well rival possession of the *jinshi* degree in terms of real power and social usefulness."[11] There were, however, also tensions brought about by all the social and economic changes in society. This was illustrated by several riots that erupted during this period, such as the silk weaver's riot in 1601, the examination riot of 1603, and the anti-eunuch riot of 1626.[12]

Suzhou in late imperial China was noted for its wealth and extravagant lifestyles. It was also one of the most populous cities, renowned for its silk production as well as for its status as the center of cultural and intellectual activities. Suzhou's cultural refinement and intellectual dominance in late imperial times has been well illustrated by scholars working in the field.[13]

Similarly, the rise and growing prosperity of Suzhou within the Lower Yangzi macroregion has been well documented by recent scholarship.[14] However, less attention has been paid to Suzhou as a major center of medical discourse. And yet, late imperial sources provide evidence of an impressive assembly of elite physicians in the region. It was also home to a lively discourse in medicine.

As early as the thirteenth century, Marco Polo had already commented on the physicians in the city of Suzhou, saying that "They have among them many physicians of great skill, who can determine the nature of a disorder and know how to apply the proper remedies."[15] Wang Wei of the Ming also commented that "I have noticed that recently when one speaks of physicians, there is no place more flourishing than Wuzhong."[16] The number of practitioners in Suzhou not only was keeping pace with the growth in population, but the significant growth of the number of physicians in the sources indicated that more elites were choosing medicine as a profession. This was due not only to a narrowing of chances for an official career, but also to a shift in attitude towards making different career choices.

Compared to the Song (960–1279) and Yuan (1264–1368) times, the number of physicians in Suzhou increased dramatically during the Ming and Qing. There seemed to have been a decline, however, from the 1600s, possibly due to unstable conditions and a downturn in the economic prosperity of the region. The establishment of the Qing dynasty and a return of political and economic stability in the region brought about a resurgence in medical activities. In local gazetteers, dynastic histories, medical treatises and biographies, we find records of three physicians in the Tang, four in the Song, five in the Yuan, eighty-eight in the Ming and two hundred and nineteen in the Qing.[17]

These figures cannot be taken as inclusive of all medical practitioners. They represented only the "sanctioned" elite of the medical community, excluding those who provided much of the health care for the common people: folk healers, midwives, religious healers, bonesetters, and the itinerant herb peddlers. Nevertheless it is an indication of the general trend of an expansion in the community of physicians in the region, and more importantly, that more members of the elite were engaging in medical activities.

Among the two hundred and nineteen physicians in the Qing, as far as can be determined, one hundred and fifty (68%) of them do not mention close family members who also practiced medicine. Of the remaining sixty-nine physicians who have immediate family members or relatives who practiced medicine, thirty-four have identifiable family members at least one-generation above who practiced medicine. The other thirty-five have records of sons or grandsons who have carried on the family tradition as a physician. It is an indication therefore that the majority of the elite physicians in the Qing did not come from families of physicians, as was commonly perceived, but that they entered into the profession through a career choice.

Although population figures recorded by officials are less than accurate, scholars have estimated that in 1229 the population in China was a little above one hundred million, and in Suzhou it was about 300,000.[18] Population increased continuously in late imperial Jiangnan. During the Ming and Qing times, Miyazaki estimates that the population in Suzhou could not have been less than one million,[19] and Mote also believes that the pre-Taiping population in Suzhou was probably close to one million.[20] Skinner however is more conservative and estimates that in 1840 population in Suzhou was probably only 700,000.[21] These figures are all lower than the numbers recorded in the local gazetteers in Suzhou. The increase in population brought about dramatic changes within the city itself, in which there was a fundamental restructuring of the core beginning in the fifteenth-century.[22]

This increase in population in Suzhou had undoubtedly brought about changes in the society and could be reflected in the dramatic lament of the eighteenth century scholar who compiled the local gazetteer:

> The country has been peaceful for a long time, and the population is a hundred times more than before. No soil on the ground is left unfarmed, no waves in the water is left un-fished, no trees and stones on the mountains are left un-gathered, yet ultimately they are insufficient to provide for the use of the people. [They become] merchants or traders, traveling to the four corners, and [among] the hundred kinds of craftsmen, the people from Wu account for the most numerous, yet often as if insufficient. Places previously without people are now filled with houses. The danger of over population has reached an extreme.[23]

The author of the gazetteer attested to not only the dramatic increase in population in the early Qing period, but a growing diversity in population as well. This diversity included an increasing number of people who took up the practice of medicine. The group of physicians in late imperial Suzhou included scholars turned physician, families of physicians, and other folk practitioners. These physicians mainly consisted of people native to Suzhou but also included people who were attracted to the area because of its dynamic medical culture.

Physicians in Suzhou

This dramatic increase in the number of physicians can arguably be attributed to a response to the rise in population in Jiangnan and a resulting expanded need for health care. But more importantly, the increase in population also meant that competition for the examinations was more severe. The Japanese scholar Miyazaki Ichisada has estimated that in the Ming and Qing, approximately one in three thousand was lucky enough to pass the examinations to reach the highest level of *jinshi* (Metropolitan Graduate).[24] Although Jiangsu and Zhejiang dominated the ranks of *jinshi* in the country,[25] the chances for success were still slim when the population figures are taken into consideration. The prevalence of failure to pass higher level examinations i.e., provincial level and up, among these physicians attests to the keen competition at the higher levels of the examination system.

The most difficult was the passing of the *juren* (Provincial Graduate) examination, which caused many scholars to abandon their studies after repeated failures and to take up medicine, a profession that allowed them to retain the ideological linkage with the scholar-official class and moral superiority over the common people. For example Zhou Yangjun, a *fugongsheng* (tribute student, second class), never was able to pass the *juren* examination and finally gave up when he was close to forty. This was also the case for Lei Dasheng who failed in the 1736 examinations, turned to medicine, and became famous for the making of pills and powders. Among the Suzhou physicians, Miao Zunyi stood out as an exception as one who passed the *jinshi* examination in 1737, but gave up an official career to take care of his ill mother.

These physicians chose to heal the biological body instead of the social body. Population increase meant that competition in the civil service examinations—the traditional path towards political, social, and economic advancement—became much more difficult. The drastic increase in the number of elite physicians, many of whom had failed repeatedly in the civil service examinations, reflected the difficulty of seeking an official career and the choice of medicine as a means of livelihood.

This increase in the number of would-be scholars turned physicians is confirmed by physicians at the time. In the preface to his *Zhangshi yitong* (Zhang's Treatise on General Medicine), published in 1695, Zhang Lu (1617–1700) discerned three major changes in medical practice, and one of them was that "since the time of the Kangxi reign (1662–1722), many Confucian scholars and gentlemen have often lowered their ambitions to become physicians. Those gentlemen who are fond of medicine regularly exchanged ideas with each other, so that their reputations became well-known for a time. Therefore medicine greatly flourished. Every household [has someone who is a] physician, this is another change in the [way of] medicine"[26]

From his account, Zhang Lu thus attested to not only an increasing trend among the scholars to give up their quests for an official career to become physicians, but that these physicians also began to form a network through which they exchanged ideas. It was through these networks they formed with each other that works were publicized and reputations made. They utilized this network in their self-fashioning as the legitimate authority in the field of medicine and medical discourse. Since power was very much associated with classical knowledge, moral virtues, and artistic tastes, their familiarity with classical knowledge and professions of benevolence in their practice enabled them to enhance their power. The state provided social legitimation for them in the form of biographical accounts included in the gazetteers and histories.

These scholars-turned-physicians were prominent in the practice of medicine in late imperial Suzhou, although they by no means dominated the medical scene. Many of Suzhou's more famous physicians and more prolific writers of medical treatises were failed examination candidates and Zhang Lu himself, coming from a family of officials, took up medicine after repeated failures in the examination. Others such as You Cheng, and You Yi (?–1749) shared a similar experience. Nevertheless, those who took up medicine were, according to Zhang Lu, considered to have "lowered their ambitions." Medicine had always been considered as the *xiaodao* (the lesser Way)[27] and choosing medicine as a career was taken as a "lowering" of one's ambitions.

This common experience in the background of many of the physicians provided them with a sense of shared identity. Furthermore, the training in the examination curriculum laid the foundation for the formation of a common bond among these examination candidates-turned-physicians. Their shared ideological and epistemological training provided a framework within which they negotiated the boundaries of medical practice.

Jiangnan not only produced many physicians of its own, it also attracted physicians from other areas of the country. Suzhou prefecture especially was attractive to many who wanted to practice medicine, due as much to its flourishing medical activities as to its being the cultural and intellectual center of late imperial China. Among the two hundred and nineteen Qing physicians mentioned in the sources in Suzhou, twelve were from other areas who moved into Suzhou and seven who for various reasons did not practice in Suzhou city.

Table 1 Suzhou City Physicians from Other Areas

Physician	native place
Feng Xie	Wujiang, Suzhou
Ye Gui	She xian, Anhui
Xu Guoqi	Jinze,Shanghai
Lu Zhenming	She xian, Anhui--to Hangzhou,Zhejiang
Wang Guangjue	She xian, Anhui
Zou Bin	Lin Tao, Lanzhou
Zheng Renyuan	Kunshan, Suzhou
Gao Ziyuan	Qiantang, Zhejiang
Shen Shiyu	Huating, Songjiang
Wei Litong	Boxiang , Zhili
Yu Zonghai	Yunjian, Songjiang
Tu Xuan	Wucheng, Zhejiang

Table 2 Suzhou Physicians Practicing Elsewhere

Physician	place of practice
Shen Laiheng	Songjiang
Li Yuchun	Shanghai
Lu Song	Zhenjiang
Lu Maoxiu	Shanghai ,Beijing
Chen Chuanzhuo	Yangzhou
Mr. Zhou	Loujiang
Zhao Rujin	Shanghai

Sources: CZXZ, MGWXZ, WXZ, YHXZ, JSLDYRZ

With the exception of Ye Gui whose family had moved to Suzhou several generations ago, and that of Wang Guangjue whose father Wang Yinglong moved the family from Anhui Shexian to Suzhou, the other physicians, as far as the sources can tell, were recent migrants. These newcomers chiefly came from the surrounding areas. She county in Anhui province was well known for its merchants and book publishing. Many of the works published were medical books and it had by this time become a major center for the publication of works in medicine. The movement into and from Suzhou was very much confined to the Jiangnan area. Lu Maoxiu had originally moved to Shanghai but went to the capital after his son Runxiang passed the highest examination and was appointed to office in the capital. The medical community in Suzhou was thus not an insular one, there were webs of connections with others. The highly commercialized nature of late imperial society, the relative convenience of transportation, and the ever-expanding world of the printed word made it a community that was served to tie the community together. It was also these networks that provided the stimulus for the lively discourse that characterized the medical community in Suzhou.

Medical practitioners in Suzhou were a diverse group. Aside from the group of scholars-turned-physicians discussed in the previous section, another group of physicians who stand out prominently in the various sources are the physicians who came from families which had practiced medicine, some of them going back several generations. Many of these physicians were well-known in Suzhou and in the Jiangnan region in general. Some of them such as Ye Gui had also studied the classics in preparation for the civil service examinations but for various reasons decided to continue with the family tradition of engaging in medical practice and often ended up with lucrative careers. This also enabled them to finance their sons' education and some had sons who passed the examinations to become officials. The very fact that these hereditary physicians also engaged in classical studies attested to the power associated with classical knowledge. It not only supplied a route to political power through the examinations, but it could also be translated into social and intellectual power and was an important factor in status formation in late imperial Chinese society. Even though it was more common for the sons to follow in the footsteps of the father to become physicians, classical education was often provided to enhance the social status of the individual as well as that of the family.

This training in the classics also meant that the hereditary physicians came to share what Bourdieu calls a "habitus" with the Confucians and the Confucian physicians.[28] Their education in the Confucian classics as well as in the medical classics, together with their practical experiences in medicine, enabled them to participate in the medical discourse on ethics and legitimacy. However, at the same time, the need for specialized medical knowledge through accumulated practical experience was acknowledged.

Approximately twenty of the recorded Qing physicians could trace at least three generations of medical practitioners within the family. Many of the hereditary physicians whose families had practiced medicine for several generations specialized in one field. For example Ye Gui's, whose medical lineage can be traced back to his grandfather Ye Shi, specialized in pediatric medicine. It was said that only after Ye Gui studied under Suzhou physician Wang Zijie did he become more adept in other fields as well.

The categories of the so-called hereditary and Confucian physicians are however sometimes misleading.[29] The terms such as *ruyi* (Confucian physician), *shiyi* (hereditary physician), *mingyi* (illustrious physician), *shiyi* (opportunist physician), *yongyi* (incompetent physician), can be found in the writings of scholars and physicians. However they reflect more the perception of the character of the physician rather than skill and ability.

The lines between these categories were also sometimes blurred by the changes the physician families experience over time. Consider the case of Zhang Lu, who studied the classics and took up medicine after repeated failures in the examinations. He came from a family of officials and his grandfather was a prominent official. He could be considered a Confucian physician but both of his sons Zhang Zhuo, and Zhang Deng, also became physicians and their status as Confucian physician is more ambiguous.

The proliferation of physicians in late imperial China and the influx of scholars into the group undoubtedly brought about anxiety among the ranks of physicians. In the absence of state regulation, control for ascendancy was mainly achieved through labeling, defining qualifications of an ideal physician, and moral constraints. The late Ming physician Xiao Jing provided one of the most elaborate categorization of physicians, he divided them into thirteen different categories: *mingyi* (illustrious physician), *ruyi* (Confucian physician), *yinyi* (secluded physician), *deyi* (virtuous physician), *shiyi* (hereditary physician), *liuyi* (itinerant physician), *sengyi* (monk physician), *mingyi* (name physician), *shiyi/yongyi* (quack physician/incompetent physician), *jianyi* (devious physician), *yinyi* (immoral physician), *nuyi* (female physician), *and yangyi* (wounds and skin infection physician).[30]

The criteria for this classification was based upon Confucian morality, although Xiao was careful to state that not all Confucians can become physicians. He nevertheless made Confucian values an important criteria in the assessment of physicians. This is not surprising in view of the fact that the author Xiao Jing himself was an aspiring Confucian who had studied for the civil service examinations and took up medicine when he was cured of a chronic illness by a famous physician.

The effort at categorization was less an attempt at systematization than the reiteration of the supremacy of Confucian ideas in medicine by a particular group of physicians. Medical discourse was mostly dominated by this elite group of physicians. They were joined by the literati, many of whom possessed medical knowledge through the reading of classical medical texts and because medicine was considered a necessary part of the training of a Confucian and an expression of moral virtue.

The labels used in the categorization were also expressions of efforts of control over the membership within the group. By using the categories, the Confucian physicians were simultaneously asserting their dominance and acknowledging the inclusion of the others into the group, even though they expressed great disdain for those without moral virtues. It was similarly a recognition of the diversity within the profession of medicine. However as we have seen in the case of Zhang Lu, the boundaries were by no means rigid, and there was considerable fluidity especially between the Confucian physicians and hereditary physicians.

Book Publishing and Emergence of Identity as a Community: The *Wuyi Huijiang* (Collected Discourses of Suzhou Physicians)

The formation of a network among the Suzhou physicians was facilitated by the emergence of a flourishing book trade and boom in publishing in the Jiangnan area. This was accompanied by a wider readership interested not only in classical literary writings, but also almanacs, practical manuals concerning things such as letter writing and medicine. This enabled the physicians not only to communicate their ideas with other physicians and scholars more efficiently, but also to extend their influence through the publication of medical primers.

This booming trade in book publishing and book markets was sustained by the highly commercialized and monetarized society in Jiangnan during the late imperial period. the growth in the printing industry probably began during the latter part of the Ming and flourished through the Qing.[31] The printing of books proliferated both under government sponsorship, such as the production of numerous encyclopedias, and through private initiatives, including private book collectors who were mainly scholars and book-sellers who printed books for profit.[32]

This vibrant book trade and book printing took on particular significance in a society which saw the erosion of traditional markers of social status as it became highly commercialized and the lines between the scholar-gentry and merchant classes became fluid. Books came to symbolize new social status in late imperial China. Dorothy Ko comments that "heightened competition for social status increased the demand for books, both as ammunition and as token of victory. It was this new market for practical instruction that fueled the commercial publishing industry and created a distinct feature of the emerging reading public."[33]

When one looks at the medical field, the dramatic increase in the number of physicians is accompanied by a similarly impressive increase in the voluminous publication of medical treatises, medical primers, and the proliferation of various genre of medical publications. Scholars have documented a thriving book trade in medical works and in the voluminous printings of collectanea of medical writings, casebooks of famous physicians, primers for the general public, and *yihua* (discourse on medicine) beginning in the mid-Ming. The following Table illustrates the increase in the publication of medical works during the Ming, and particularly the Qing.

From the table it is clear that there was a dramatic increase in book production during the Ming and Qing in Jiangsu. This surge in written medical works corresponded to the increase in the number of physicians in this area during this period. Written works served not only to consolidate the position of a profession which was just establishing itself and enabled the elite physicians to validate their reputations through publications, but it also enabled them to exert control. This was particularly important for the elite physicians who had only recently come onto the scene and thus had to compete with the hereditary physicians to establish their legitimacy. This effort played out particularly in debates over the issue of “three generations” and the place of Zhang Zhongjing (Chapter One). Experience had always been an important factor in the selection of a physician as revealed in proverbs such as: "Old physician, young shaman." (*laoyi shaobu*. Traditionally, it had been believed that the best physicians came from a family of at least three generations. The motto from *Liji* (Book of Rites) that "one does not take the medicine of the physician who did not come from three generations" (*yibusanshi bufuqiyao*) serves to illustrate this ideal. It is not surprising that this became one of the most contentious discussions among the physicians.

Written works not only enabled the physicians to express their ideas but served as a form of evaluation and criteria of competence. Thus the hereditary physician achieved their reputations and legitimacy through generations of practicing physicians, while these Confucian physicians who had newly entered the field, and could not claim accumulated wisdom passed down from their

Table 3 Medical Works by Jiangsu Physicians

	Pre-Song	Song	Yuan	Ming	Qing	Total
1. *yijing*	2	0	0	15	60	77
(yunqi)						
2. *zhenfa*	0	3	0	19	38	60
3. *shanghan*	1	8	1	7	183	220
(*jinkui*						
wenbing)						
4. *bencao*	6	1	0	19	68	94
5. *zhenjiu*	0	1	2	10	12	25
6. *fanglun*						
neike	26	8	10	121	336	501
waike	0	3	0	15	31	49
fuke	0	0	0	8	25	33
erke	0	2	0	33	56	91
yanke	0	0	1	7	5	13
houke	0	0	0	1	11	13
7. *yishi*	0	0	0	18	160	178
(*yian*						
yihua)						
8. *yangsheng*	1	0	0	5	22	28
9. *tuina*	0	0	0	0	7	7
10.*zalu*	0	1	0	6	54	61

*Data compiled from Guo Aichun, *Zhongguo Fensheng Yijikao* (A Study of Medical Works in China According to Provinces) vol.1 (Tianjin: Tianjin Kexue Jishu Chubanshe, 1984), pp. 401–818.

forefathers, established their legitimacy and spread their reputation through writing medical treatises.

It was also through these written medical works that a network of communication was set up which facilitated a growing group consciousness. The publication of these materials in addition served to formulate guidelines for the conduct and practice of medicine, directly challenging the long-held tradition of selecting a physician based upon his "three generations" of practical experience. One of the most dramatic increases was in the *yishi* (history of medicine) category which included the *yian* (medical cases) and *yihua* (conversations in medicine). Publication in this category during the Qing accounted for almost 90% of the total publications in Jiangsu. Another category which showed dramatic increase included works on *shanghan* (cold damaged disorders) and *wenbing* (heat factor disorders), reflecting a growing interest especially during the late Ming and Qing in treatments of epidemics.

The largest book trade centers in Jiangsu province during the Ming and Qing were Nanjing and Suzhou. In Suzhou most of the book trade was concentrated outside of Changmen in the fashionable northwestern part of the city of Wuxian. The largest center of publication of medical works was in Huizhou, Xinan. Suzhou physicians were active participants in the boom of medical publishing. It was also through these publications that the physicians formed a social and intellectual network.

Among the *Yixue congshu* (medical collectanea), Zhang Lu's *Zhangshi yitong* (Zhang's Treatise on General Medicine) was one of the most famous. *Congshu* generally "provided a medium by which Chinese scholar-printers could publish or reprint their rare books, as well as short works of scholarship and newly collated versions of previously published texts."[34] Zhang's work was published in 1695 and in his preface he lamented the situation in medicine in his times. His stated goal was to publish his work so that others who wanted to learn medicine could use it as a guide. This undoubtedly was useful for many of the failed examination candidates who needed to learn medicine. Zhang Lu's work was attractive to them not only because of the practical guidance, but also due to the familiarity of the language used, and the moral exhortation to be a benevolent physician, providing justification for their choice of career.

Interest in medicine was not just limited to the physicians and the Confucian elite. There was also widespread interest in medicine on the part of the general public. Publication of primers proliferated, written by the elite physicians for the general reading public, primers contained ideas and methods written in a way that was easy to memorize and recite. The primers written by Fujian physician Chen Nianzu (1766–1833)[35] were widely circulated.[36] As a result, classical knowledge in medicine no longer was the prerogative of the elite. These primers circulated not only circulated technical medical knowledge but also the values of the elite physicians. The politics of knowledge were, however, more complex. As Roy Porter pointed out, "Popularization could be part of the tactics of a 'professional medicine', itself but shakily established, attempting to assert its own superiority; or it could serve as a weapon against it."[37] While popularization of this kind of medical knowledge extended their influence, it also allowed others to challenge their authority.

Physicians frequently "borrowed" the names of more famous physicians to lend legitimacy and popularity to their works.[38] For example Chen Nianzu used the name of Ye Tianshi when he first published his *Yixue congzhonglu* (Record of Medicine for the Masses) but later stated that he wished to *shouhui* (take it back) and have it published under his own name.[39] This practice was apparently quite popular among the literati as well. Among the physicians, it seems that the name of Ye Tianshi was popularly "borrowed", attesting to his reputation and popularity.

Zhang Lu's comments on changes in the medical scene discussed above attest to the fact that more scholars were abandoning their studies to become physicians. At the same time, there was a lively forum of medical discourse amongst the physicians who apparently communicated frequently with each other and lauded each other's works. It was part of the self-fashioning of their legitimacy and superiority in medicine. The friends and the networks which they set up were the best resources they had in the quest for legitimation in the field of medicine and elevation of social status.

Two works in Suzhou further illustrate the emerging consciousness of the Suzhou physicians as a community. During the Kangxi period, there was the collection of medical cases *Wuzhong yian* (A Collection of Medical Cases from Suzhou) by Guo Yizhi. The other is the collection of medical essays, the *Wuyi huijiang* (Collected Discourses of Suzhou Physicians, hereafter cited as WYHJ) by Tang Dalie, a physician who was active during the Qianlong and Jiaqing reigns. Both of these took Suzhou as their geographical location.

Guo Yizhi's *Wuzhong yiani* was listed in the *yiwen* section of MGWXZ[40] and there was a preface written by Huang Zhongjian that is still available. The work itself, however, is no longer extant. It is from Tang Dalie's preface to his own *Wuyi huijiang* that we know Guo's work was a collection of medical cases of physicians during the Kangxi reign.[41] Guo was a physician of considerable fame and practiced medicine in Guangfu li (Guangfu town). From Huang Zhongjian's preface to Guo's work we are told that although Guo practiced medicine and had become quite famous, he never gave up on his classical studies and still had aspirations for an official career. When Huang visited him, he found on Guo's desk the books he studied for the *juye* (civil service examination).[42] Unfortunately, we do not know which medical cases were collected and the criteria that were employed to select the cases.

Guo's work inspired Tang Dalie to edit the *Wuyi huijiang* and collect the writings of forty-one authors, totaling one hundred and forty-three essays. Most scholars in China consider the WYHJ the first medical journal published in traditional China. Recently, Fu Weikang in *Zhongguo yixueshi* (A History of Medicine in China) comments that the WYHJ was edited from 1792 to 1801, the year Tang died, and published a total of eleven *juan*.[43] It has been speculated that one *juan* was published each year to make up the total of eleven.[44] Recently scholars have voiced doubt as to whether it was actually a medical journal. In a recent article, Su Tiege examines the various different editions that were published and concludes that the WYHJ was not a medical journal published in consecutive years as many had thought; rather it was a collection of medical essays.[45] Su, however, does not discussed the significance of the 1814 edition, which was edited by Tang Dalie's grandson Qingqi.

Tang Dalie, in his *WYHJ*, provided explanatory notes concerning the publication of materials in the collection. I have translated them in their entirety despite the length because it not only sheds light on the publication of medical works during the early Qing period, and the networks forming among the physicians, but it also gives insights into some of the customs and problems in the world of publication in late imperial Jiangnan.

Fanli[46] (Explanatory Notes)

1. This collection will include all essays, regardless of whether it is a specialization in internal, external, women, or pediatric medicine, that have interesting stories concerning medicine, found what previous people never found, and writings that can contribute to people's learning. For those which repeat what other have said, we will not reprint what is already abundant in previous works.
2. Each gentleman should put before each piece their names, noting posthumous names, ranks and native places. If it is an old manuscript by their forefathers, then the year of birth and death should also be noted, and that it was asked that descendent (name) publish it. This is to imitate the idea of short biographies. They should also be on separate sheets, so that they are not connected, so as to facilitate adding supplements.
3. Whenever you honor us with your eminent essays, they will be printed as they are received. There will be no categorization and no limit on the

length. The order of publication will not be based upon the age of the author, nor will it be ranked according to the order it was received. It is hoped that the essays will increase steadily, and become something worth reading. If your honorable home is far away, it does not matter to send to my humble hut through post, so that it can be printed

4. Everyone's inclinations are different. Collecting different people's writings in a book will unavoidably find differences of opinions among the works. If one is preserved and the other discarded, I am afraid that it is like immobilizing one's eyes, it is not amassing discussions. If each can penetrate a principle, then it does not matter to take both views, and let the reader choose. This is also a way of expanding learning.
5. This collection is to gather all colleagues' (*tongxue*)[47] discourse on what they have learned in their studies, analyzing the doubtful and appreciating the wonderful. They do not appropriate the platitudes of old scholars. If there seems to be antiquated words in glancing, by looking at the places where they espouse their meanings, there will be words which are different and original. It is only because by narrating from the beginning, they cannot avoid quoting old texts for assistance, it must not be seen as plagiarizing.
6. For the essays in this collection, there are eloquently written ones, and there are also ones that are absolutely vulgar. It is for each to suit their own inclinations, as long as they get their meanings across. Even though the writing is ridiculed, the essence can be passed on.
7. Whenever a new book is published, the bookstores often immediately reprint it. Although it is said that it will be investigated, this abuse has been going on for a long time. This collection of mine is published according to whoever first offers his works, and now it is also advertised widely, so that even my own unworthy writing is included, the accumulation is quite substantial. Now because the (chapters) are unbalanced, therefore I will first print several, then wait until colleagues gradually grant their opinions. I will also gradually print according to order. These several chapters do not make a finished book. Those who buy and read this should know the original edition of this (tang), so that chapters can be added day by day. As for the reprints, how can they be reprinted and augmented at the same time, it is definitely not the whole collection, we wish all people to carry this out.[48]

These directions and regulations are quoted at length here because Tang Dalie's publication of the WYHJ indicated acceptance of a forum for the different physicians and scholars to publish their ideas. Tang's emphasized tolerating diversity in medical discourse and accepting writings that presented good and original ideas. In doing so he took aim at those well-educated physicians who could compose eloquent prose and write in style, but did not tolerate physicians who were not as well educated and were unable to frame their ideas so eloquently. It was an example of the use of classical training as a means of differentiation among the physicians. The two groups of physicians were distinguished from each other by their education in the Confucian classics, but linked together in their knowledge and practice of medicine. The practice of medicine was a common factor which bound them together in a shared consciousness and identity. It is apparent that there were some physicians who were not as well-trained in scholarship were also participating in the discourse. Tang Dalie indicated that there were "vulgar" writings, meaning that they were not as elegant, but implored others to accept them and focus on the ideas rather than the style of writing.

Tang not only called for the tolerance of different styles of writing and levels of sophistication, but also asked for the acceptance of different views. This attests to a growing divergence of opinions among physicians in the region. This can be attributed the growing number of physicians, and to the increasing tendency to question existing ways of healing and prescriptions. Waves of epidemics also challenged conventional methods of healing and stimulated new ways of thinking.

There is also a hint of egalitarianism in Tang's Preface in his assertion that all essays will be printed and that they will not be ranked, even according to age. This reflects the increasing fluidity in social status as the region experienced a flourishing economy and changes in traditional social stratification and hierarchy. All social strata, all opinions were welcomed and Tang vowed in his Preface to print essays that he received. The boundaries between Confucian and hereditary physicians especially appears blurred here.

Tang's preface suggests that medical practice was dominated by several fields of specialization: internal and external medicine, children (pediatrics), and women (gynecology, obstetrics). These specializations in medicine represented a kind of specialized knowledge that was mainly passed down through family traditions in which the accumulation of experience was emphasized. Most of the physicians in these specialized fields came from families who had practiced medicine for several generations and had therefore built up a reputation in the region. These were the physicians that the Confucian physicians were attempting to compete with, leading some to argue that it was not family tradition (three practicing generations), but learning through books (three medical classics) that should be the basis of judgment of a good physician.

Tang's work reveals the problem of "stealing" publications in late imperial China.[49] Tang did caution that not all references to other works could be considered plagiarism. It was, nevertheless, a serious problem that plagued both the publishing of medical works and other literary works.

We can see that book collecting and printing were actively undertaken by scholars in the Jiangnan region.[50] These efforts contributed to the dissemination of medical knowledge and the creation of a network of literary communication among scholars and physicians in the Jiangnan region. Works such as the WYHJ provided a forum for the exchange of ideas among the different groups of physicians, attesting to a lively medical scene.

Notes

[1] During the Qin dynasty (221–207 B.C.) it was transformed into Kuaiji prefecture *(jun)* and later the Sui elevated it to a *zhou* and renamed it Suzhou after the Gusu mountains in the region. The Song (960–1126) further elevated it as the Pingjiang *fu* with six counties and under the Yüan it became the Pingjiang *lu* (circuit).

[2] In the Ming the seven counties were: Wuxian, Changzhou, Qunshan, Changshu, Wujiang, Jiading, Chongming. In the Qing the nine counties were: Wuxian, Changzhou, Yuanhe, Qunshan, Xinyang, Changshu, Zhaowen, Wujiang, Chenze.

[3] The influx of people from outside of Suzhou can be attested to by the setting up of numerous guilds, *huiguan*, which mostly grouped together merchants or craftsmen from the same native place. For example the Jiangxi *huiguan*, set up in 1648, looked after the needs of merchants in different trades from Jiangxi as well as provided care for officials from Jiangxi. Beginning from the mid-Qing however, the trend shifted towards the setting up of *gongsuo*, which emphasized trade rather than the same native place. There were about 114 *gongsuo* in Suzhou during the Qing. See Xu Dixin and Wu Chengming, *Zhongguo zibenchuyi di mengya* (Beijing: Renmin chubanshe, 1985) pp. 296–306.

[4] See John Lossing Buck, *Land Utilization in China* (Nanking: The University of Nanking, 1937) and also *Science and Civilization in China*, vol.6, part 2, by Francesca Bray (Cambridge: Cambridge University Press, 1984).

[5] In other versions Huzhou is replaced by Changzhou, but the centrality of Suzhou remains unchanged.

[6] Philip C.C. Huang, *The Peasant Family and Rural Development in the Yangzi Delta, 1350–1988* (Stanford: Stanford University Press, 1990). Wu Chengming, *Zhongguo ibenzhuyi de mengya* (The Sprouting of Capitalism in China), vol.1 of *Zhongguo zibenzhuyi fazhan shi* (The History of the Development of Capitalism in China). (Beijing: Xinhua shudian, 1985).

[7] Susan Naquin and Evelyn S. Rawski, *Chinese Society in the Eighteenth Century* (New Haven: Yale University Press, 1987), p. 100.

[8] *Ming Qing Suzhou Gongshangye beikeji*. (Jiangsu: Renmin chubanshe, 1981).

[9] Peng Xingwei, *Zhongguo huobishi* (History of Currency in China) (Shanghai: Shanghai Renmin Chubanshe, 1988).

[10] Joseph Esherick and Mary Rankin ed., *Chinese Local Elites and Patterns of Dominance* (Berkeley: University of California Press, 1990), p.20.

[11] Cynthia Browkaw, *The Ledgers of Merit and Demerit: Social Change and Moral Order in Late Imperial China* (Princeton: Princeton University Press, 1991), p. 6.

[12] For more details on the riots, see Tsing Yuan, "Urban Riots and Disturbances" in *From Ming to Ch'ing: Conquest, Region, and Continuity in Seventeenth-Century China* ed. by Jonathan D. Spence and John E. Wills, Jr. (New Haven: Yale University Press, 1979), pp. 279–320. See also Fuma Susumu's discussion on Hangzhou in " Late Ming Urban Reform and Popular Uprising in Hangzhou" in *Cities of Jiangnan in Late Imperial China*, pp. 47–79.

[13] For example see Benjamin Elman, *From Philosophy to Philology: Intellectual and Social Aspects of Change in Late Imperial China* (Cambridge: Harvard University Press, 1984) and *Classicism, Politics, and Kinship: The Ch'ang-Chou School of New Text Confucianism in Late Imperial China* (Berkeley: University of California Press, 1990).

[14] See for example Duan Benluo and Zhang Qifu, *Suzhou Shougongyeshi* (History of Handicraft Industries in Suzhou) (Jiangsu: Jiangsu Guji chubanshe, 1986). Fan Jinmin "Qing Qianqi Suzhou nongye jingji di tese" (The Characteristics of Agricultural Economy in Suzhou during the Early Qing) in *Zhongguo nongshi* (Chinese Agriculture), 12:1 (1993): 46–51. Hong Huanchun, "Lun Ming Qing Suzhou Diqu Huiguan de Xingzhi ji qi zuoyong" (A Discussion on the Nature and Uses of Local Guilds in Suzhou during the Ming and Qing) in *Zhongguoshi yanjiu* (Study of Chinese History) 1980, no.2: 3–15. Michael Marmê, "Heaven on Earth: The Rise of Suzhou, 1127–1550" in *Cities in Jiangnan in Late Imperial China*, ed. by Linda Cooke Johnson (New York: State University of New York Press, 1993), pp. 17–45. Paolo Santangelo, "Urban Society in Late Imperial Suzhou" in ibid., pp. 81–116. Hiroshi Ihara *Soshu* (Suzhou) (Tokyo: Kôdansha, 1993). Miyazaki Ichisada, "Mingshin jidai no Soshu to keikogyo no hattatsu" (The Development of Light Industries in Suzhou during the Ming and Qing) in *Miyazaki Ichisada zenshû* (The Complete Works of Miyazaki Ichisada), vol.13, (Tokyo: Iwanami Shoten, 1992), pp.80–93.

[15] *The Travels of Marco Polo*, ed. by Milton Rugoff (New York: New American Library, 1986), p. 182.

[16] Wuzhong refers to Wu *xian* and the surrounding areas. Quotation from Wang Wei "Lun Yi" (Discourse on Physicians) in *Gujin tushu jicheng.yibu quanlu* (Collection of Works Past and Present: Complete Collection of the Medical Section) 518:434.

[17] Based on tabulation in CZWXZ (*Chongzhen wuxian zhi, Gazetteer of Wu county compiled in the Chongzhen reign)* MGWXZ (*Mingguo wuxian zhi*, Gazetteer of Wu country, compiled during the Republican era), SZFZ,GSZ (*Gusu zhi*, *Gazetteer of the Gusu region)* CZXZ (*Changzhou xian shi*, Gazetteer of Changzhou county),QLSZFZ, MS (*Mingshi*, History of the Ming Dynasty), QSG (*Qingshigao*, Draft of Qing Dynasty History), WYHJ (*Wuyi huijiang*, Collected Discourses of Suzhou Physicians). These figures come close to what Chen Daojin and Xue Weitao have estimated in *Jiangsu Lidai Yirenzhi* (Collection of Jiangsu Physicians from Successive Dynasties) (Jiangsu: Jiangsu kexue jishu chubanshe, 1985).

[18] Mote's estimate of Suzhou's population, although it seems somewhat high. See Frederick Mote, "A Millennium of Chinese Urban History: Form, Time, and Space Concepts in Soochow" in *Rice University Studies*, 59.4 (1973): 35–65.

[19] Miyazaki Ichisada, "Soshu to Yangshu" in *Miyazaki Ichisada zenshû*. pp.375–376.

[20] Mote, 1973: p. 39.

[21] Skinner, 1977, p.29.

[22] Michael Marmê, "Population and Possibility in Ming (1368–1644) Suzhou: A Quantified Model," in *Ming Studies* 12 (Spring 1981): 29–64. Marmê looks at the changes in the core and periphery and challenges Mote's presentation of an unchanging Suzhou in his now famous juxtaposition of the 1229 *Pingjiang tubei* and the 1945 aerial photo.

[23] Qianlong Wuxianzhi, *juan* 5 as quoted in Hong Huanchun, *Ming Qing Suzhou nongcun jingji zhiliao* (Materials on the Economy of Suzhou Villages in the Ming and Qing) (Suzhou: Jiangsu guji chubanshe, 1988), p. 646.

[24] Miyazaki Ichisada: *Chûgoku no shiken jigoku* (The Civil Service Examinations: China's Examination Hell) 1963 first edition (Tokyo: Chûô kôronsha, 1986), p.199. For a discussion on social mobility and the examination system see Ho Ping-ti, *The Ladder of Success in Imperial China* (New York: Columbia University Press, 1962).

[25] Ho Ping-ti, *The Ladder of Success in Imperial China*, pp.226–237.

[26] Zhang Lu, *Zhangshi yitong* (Zhang's Treatise on General Medicine) 1719 preface edition, (Shanghai: Shanghai kexue jishu chubanshe, 1963), p.1.

[27] Zhu Xi in his commentary on the *Analects* portrayed medicine as a *jianye* (low profession). See Unschuld's discussion on Zhu Xi in *Medical Ethics in Imperial China*, pp.38–40.

[28] Bourdieu suggests that a *habitus* should be "understood as a system of lasting, transposable dispositions which, integrating past experiences, functions at every moment as a *matrix of perceptions, and actions* and makes possible the achievement of infinitely diversified tasks." Pierre Bourdieu, *Outline of a Theory of Practice*, translated by Richard Nice (Cambridge: Cambridge University Press, 1972), pp.82–83.

[29] Officially, during the Ming, physician statuses were supposed to be hereditary. The Hongwu emperor, in an attempt to ensure a stable society, proclaimed laws that made professional status hereditary. The three categories were the *min* (commoners), *jun* (military), and *jiang* (artisan). The *min* category included the *ju* (scholars). the *yi* (medical practitioners), and the *yinyang* (geomancers). See *Mingshi*, *shihuo* 77. In 1386 a decree was also issued exhorting the four classes: *shi* (scholars), *nong* (farmers), *gong* (artisans), and *shang* (merchants), to observe their proper stations. Physicians and geomancers (*bu*) were locals and thus forbidden to travel to faraway places. However as the society experienced changes in the economy and in population, these fixed statuses became more and more difficult to maintain. See *Mingtaitsu shilu*, 177.

[30] Xiao Jing, *Xuanqi jiuzhenglun* (Discourse on Rectification According to the Yellow Emperor's Treatise) Preface 1644. (Beijing: Zhongyi guji chubanshe, 1983), pp. 509–536.

[31] For a general discussion on the shifts in printing centers in China see Nagasawa Kikuya "Shina kokon kokusho chi no hensen (Changes in the Past and Present Book Printing Places in China) 15.5, 1940: 137–140. For a discussion on publishing in Jiangnan during the late Ming see Oki Yasushi, "Minmatsu Kônan ni okeru shuppan bunka no kenkyû" (A Study of the Print Culture in Late Ming Jiangnan). *Hiroshima Daigaku bungakubu kiyô* 50, special issue no. 1 (January 1991): 1–176.

[32] For a discussion on libraries and printing in Jiangnan see Benjamin A. Elman, *From Philosophy to Philology: Intellectual and Social Aspects of Change in Late Imperial China* (Cambridge: Council on East Asian Studies, Harvard University, 1984), pp. 139–

170. Also Wei Yinru, *Zhongguo shuji yinshuashi* (The History of Book Printing in China) (Beijing: Yinshua gongye chubanshe, 1984), pp.94–198, 211–245. Liu Guojun, "Song-Yuan-Ming-Qing di keshu shiye" (The Profession of Book Printing in Song-Yuan-Ming-Qing) in *Zhongguo tushushi ziliaoji* (Collection of Materials on the History of Books in China) edited by Liu Jiabi (Hong Kong: Longmeng shudian, 1974), pp. 481–498. Shen Sheyuan, "Mingdai Jiangsu keshu shiye gaishu" (A Brief Account of the Profession of Book Publishing in Jiangsu during the Ming) in *Lidai keshu gaikuang* (Beijing: Yinshua gongye chubanshe, 1991), pp.309–317.

[33] Dorothy Ko, *Teachers of the Inner Chambers: Women and Culture in Seventeenth-Century China* (Stanford: Stanford University Press, 1994), p. 34.

[34] Elman, *From Philosophy to Philology*, p. 151. See also p. 152 for the criteria of *congshu.*

[35] Zi Xiuyuan. He studied the Classics for taking the examinations and passed the *juren* (provincial graduate) examination in 1792. He studied medicine under a physician named Cai Zongyu and practiced medicine in his spare time as a magistrate.

[36] *Yixue Congzhonglu* (Record of Medicine for the Masses) (Fuzhou: Fujian kexue jishu chubanshe, 1987) and *Yixue sanzijing* (Three-word Primer for Medicine), author preface 1804, 12th printing (Shanghai: Shanghai kexue jishu chubanshe, 1991).

[37] Roy Porter ed., *The Popularization of Medicine 1650–1850* (New York: Routledge, 1992), p.8.

[38] Barbara Volkmar's article "The Physician and the Plagiarists: The Fate of the Legacy of Wan Quan" illustrates clearly the prevalence of plagiarism and "borrowing" of names in late imperial medical publishing. In *The East Asian Library Journal*, vol. 9 no. 1 (Spring 2000): 1–77.

[39] "*Fanli*" (Explanatory Notes) in *Yixue congzhonglu* (Record of Medicine for the Masses), p.1.

[40] MGWXZ (*Mingguo Wuxian zhi*, Gazetteer of Wu County during the Republican period) 56b.

[41] WYHJ, preface, p.1.

[42] *Guangfu zhi*, 1929 edition, *juan* 11. Huang Zhongjian, *"Xianchuan douzhen qishu xu"*

[43] Fu Weikang ed. *Zhongguo yixueshi* (A History of Medicine in China) (Shanghai: Xinhua shudian, 1990), pp. 440–441.

[44] Jin Shoushan , "Woguo zuizao de yixue zazhi—Wuyi huijiang" (China's earliest medical journal—the *Wuyi huijiang*) in *Zhongyi Zazhi* (Chinese Medical Journal) 1985, 25.1: 70–71.

[45] Su Tiege, "*Wuyi huijiang* wei lianxu chuban kanwu zhi zhiyi" (On the Question of *Wuyi huijiang* as a Consecutive Publication) in *zhonghua yishi zazhi* (Chinese Medical Journal) 1993, 23.3:145–148.

[46] *Fanli* is generally a set of directions for the readers, which introduces the work and explains the plan and style of the work.

[47] *Tongxue* generally referred to those who studied under the same teacher. Here it refers to all those who have undertaken the study of medicine. It is also indicative of a sense of common bond and identity.

[48] WYHJ, *fanli* (explanatory notes).

[49] The problem of unauthorized reprinting of materials seems to be a widespread one in late imperial China and there is no lack of lamentations by scholars on this type of "stealing." For a discussion on the concept of intellectual property and the introduction of intellectual property law see William P. Alford's *To Steal a Book is An Elegant Offense:*

Intellectual Property Law in Chinese Civilization (Stanford: Stanford University Press, 1995).

[50] See Benjamin Elman, *From Philosophy to Philology*, pp. 140–159.

CHAPTER FIVE

Maintaining Health in Suzhou

THE use of the metaphor of physicians as rulers of the body and medicine as soldiers rectifying disorders not only conferred a special status upon the medical practitioners and enabled them to rise above the traditional boundaries of the artisan (*gong*), but it also imposed a moral framework upon those who ruled. The statesman and the physician were both bound by the moral obligation of *ren* (benevolence). The former was expected to display *renzheng* (benevolent rule) while the latter worked under the assumption of practicing *renshu* (benevolent craft). The ultimate goal of both the statesman and the physician was to achieve the state of *ping* (peace) and *he* (harmony) within the social and biological body respectively. The expression of benevolence for the common people and the maintenance of order and harmony within a peaceful society thus became important tasks for the ruler in his claim of the legitimacy to rule. We have seen how patronage of medicine was used by the Mongol rulers in China to express their benevolence in Chapter Two.

More important than healing, however, was prevention. For the virtuous sage, the attainment of a peaceful society, similar to the wise physician, is rooted not in the curing of ills but in prevention. Thus the *Siqi tiaoshen dalunpian* (The Expanded Discourse on Harmonizing the Spirit in the Four Seasons) *Huangdi neijing suwen* (Inner Canon of the Yellow Emperor: Basic Questions) says[1]:

> Therefore [to say] the sage does not cure the already sick [but] cures [those] not yet sick, [does not] regulate disorder that has already occurred, [but] regulates before [the occurrence] of disorder, this is the meaning. If medicine is administered after [one has already] fallen sick, regulation is carried out after disorder has occurred, [this can be] compared to like digging a well when thirsty, to cast an awl because of fighting. Is it not too late!

For the state, therefore, medicine was not only a moral responsibility to provide people with medicine and medical care during times of need such as epidemics and other disasters, but it was also a practical strategy in the maintenance of political legitimacy through the prevention of disorder by offering care to the poor and needy. The setting up of pharmacies and charitable associations provided care for the needy and a safety net for the poor.

State policy in the caring for the health of the people can be found as early as in the *Zhouli* (Rituals of Zhou) when the *jiyi* (physicians of illness) were charged with the care of the illness of the different seasons that plague the people. Whenever there was illness among the people, they were treated according to their illness. When they died the *jiyi* recorded the causes for the deaths and provided the records to the *yishi* (physician) who were responsible for the administration of medical policies.[2]

There was increasingly active government involvement in the provision of health care and the maintenance of public health beginning in the mid-Tang dynasty when the government took over the administration of charitable infirmaries for the poor such as the *Beitianfang* (Infirmary of the Grieved Fields) and the *angbingfang* (Infirmary of Nourishing the Sick) from the Buddhist monasteries after the persecution of Buddhism in 845.[3] The Tang government also set up medical administration in the provinces. In an edict issued in 723, Emperor Xuanzong decreed that "[I]n faraway districts and secluded provinces, there is a complete lack of medicine, what will the poor rely on for sickness and suffering? It should be ordered for all the provinces to each install a *yixue boshi* (medical official). Each province should place in store together with the classics and histories *bencao* (*materia medica*) collected verified prescriptions."[4] In 739 it was decreed for those provinces with more than one hundred thousand *hu* (households) to designate twenty *yisheng* (student of general medicine), those with less than one hundred thousand *hu* were to have twelve. These medical personnel were to patrol the provincial area for the treatment of illnesses.[5] The government also published medical prescriptions for the benefit of all people.[6]

The setting up of institutional networks to provide medical care for the people continued in the Song with the establishment of the *huimin yaoju* (Pharmacy for the Benefit of the People) which were continued into the Ming. They were established not just by the central government but were also set up in local areas to sell medicine at below market rate or to distribute free medicine to the poor.[7] The Song also set up medical practitioners in the provinces with seven in the provinces and one to five for counties for every ten thousand *hu* in the counties.[8]

The Song government undertook the task of extensively collecting prescriptions, compiling and publishing them for dissemination. There were several results of these efforts. In 992 the *Taiping shenghui fang* (Taiping Prescriptions of Sacred Benevolence) was published, consisting of over ten thousand prescriptions.

The Song government's efforts in attempting to collect and publish prescriptions represented not only the extension of government interest in medical practice, but it also represented a major effort at the standardization of medicine, its practice and its knowledge. These *ju fang* (Pharmacy Prescriptions) were chosen based upon the criteria of learned medicine and represented a further break between the learned and the folk traditions in medicine. These *ju fang* also became the focus of much contention later on when Confucian physicians criticized many other medical practitioners of blindly following the *ju fang* without a full understanding of the principles of medical theory.

The Yuan government continued and elaborated on the medical administration in the prefectures and counties by setting up a *tiju* (supervisor) at each *lu* (circuit) for the supervision of medical affairs. Each prefecture had physicians divided into fifteen ranks.[9]

Therefore from the Tang to the Yuan, there was increasing government involvement in the area of local medical administration. The provision of medical care not just in times of need but the setting up of regular medical offices and provision of physicians trained in the classical tradition for the care of the common people not only was a manifestation of the benevolence of the ruler, but it was part of an effort to establish a degree of conformity in the heterogeneous medical culture in traditional China. Through the distribution of medicine through pharmacies it was in effect ratifying the type of medicine that was being promoted, i.e. the learned tradition. The appointment of physicians at the prefectural and county levels and their endowment with the authority of the state elevated their statuses and the status of the classical medical tradition. It in effect ratified the learned tradition as legitimate in the practice of medicine and empowered it over the other traditions.

Medical Administration in Late Imperial Suzhou

In her study on Ming-Qing medicine in the Lower Yangzi area, Angela Leung has found increasing government retreat from the provision of medical relief in times of disasters and in medical education, accompanied by a democratization of medical knowledge.[10] The retreat of the state from the provision of local welfare is echoed by William Rowe in his study on Hankow. He has also found that although the Qing government did sponsor welfare agencies for the provision of services to the poor, "At no time did the Ch'ing state aspire to any significant role in providing a "safety net" for the downwardly mobile in Hankow society" and that it showed "a further pulling back from direct government involvement."[11]

This general sense of the withdrawal of the state and the decline of its ineffectiveness is challenged by Pierre-Etienne Will in his study on famine relief[12] and also in his study with Bin Wong on the granary system.[13] Did the government seemingly "retreat" from active promotion and intervention of the education and administration of medical care in the provinces in late imperial China? To answer this we must first look at some of the institutions that were set up by the state to promote medical affairs and state involvement in the provision of medical care at the local levels.

In 1384 the Ming government set up a *zhengke* (prefectural physician) at the *fu* (prefectural) level, a *dianke* (departmental physician) at the *zhou* (departmental) level, and a *xunke* (county physician) at the *xian* (county) level. Yet they were all low level titles,*cong jiupin* (ninth rank lower class), without compensation.[14] There were also *huimin yaoju* set up in the local districts with physicians in attendance. The Qing also set up the local medical administration after the Ming system. The physicians were certified by the *libu* (Ministry of Rites) and were under the supervision of the Provincial Administration Commission (*zhengxuan buzheng shishi*).

The setting up of a *yixue* (Medical Bureau) can be traced to the Yuan when one was set up at the northeastern corner of the county seat with sacrifices being offered to the *Sanhuang miao* (Temple of the Three Emperors).[15] In Ming Suzhou the *yixue* was built in 1562, but because it gradually fell into disrepair, it was rebuilt in the Qing during the reign of the Kangxi emperor in 1696. Later it was abandoned, although the exact date is unknown.[16] It was probably sometime in the mid-nineteenth century since it was already listed as abandoned in the Tongzhi edition of the Suzhou gazetteer.

Most of the physicians in Suzhou did not associate with the official medical academy, although as we shall see they more than willingly provided services to the special bureaus set up during times of epidemics and other disasters. There is no evidence that the medical academy in Suzhou attempted in any way to regulate the practice of medicine by the numerous physicians, nor did they attempt to dominate the transmission of medical knowledge.

One of the most famous physicians who was associated with the Suzhou district medical academy was Tang Dalie (1792–1801), compiler of the *Wuyi huijiang* (Collected discourses of Suzhou physicians). Tang Dalie (?–1801), *zi* Lisan *hao* Lisan also Lindeng, was a native of Changzhou county. He had originally studied the classics but there was no indication that he had taken any examinations. He became a *dianyuguan* (warden) and treated prisoners who were ill. Later he was appointed as Suzhou's *yixue zhengke* (Principal of the Suzhou Prefectural Medical School). He is best known for his collection and compilation of medical works in Suzhou and publishing it as the *Wuyi huijiang* (Collected Discourse of Suzhou Physicians), discussed in detail in Chapter Four. In the WYHJ he had included writings of physicians from the Suzhou district medical academy who were otherwise unmentioned in the other sources. For example, Wang Yuanshi, the Principal of Changzhou country's medical academy, Tang Xueji, principal of the Suzhou medical academy and Weng Jieshou, who had been principal of Wu county's medical academy. We know very little about these people and their backgrounds. It can be speculated that they were left out of the government sponsored sources because of their lack of connection to the learned tradition. Thus even though they were officials of the local medical academies, they were not considered as fitting the criteria for mention.

Epidemics in Suzhou

In addition to the provision of medical care for the poor and destitute through the various charitable institutions, one of the important functions of the state was to care for the people during times of epidemics. State interest in times of natural disasters and the provision of relief materials was based mainly on the desire to maintain order within society. Thus the seventeenth-century magistrate Huang Liuhong in his memoir and handbook for magistrates, written in the 1690s, comments on famine relief: "[R]elief materials are dispensed in a variety of ways. Rice-gruel kitchens can save the lives of thousands of famine victims, but famine relief should be administered with the purpose of preventing the recipients from leaving home, so that the government can retain millions of people on the tax rolls."[17]

During the late Ming and Qing, China suffered major epidemic outbreaks in the 1580s, 1640s, and 1820s.[18] These outbreaks were unparalleled in their extent and severity. Elvin estimates that "In 1588, the worst year of the first of these outbreaks, ninety-two localities (that is, prefectures or counties) in thirteen provinces suffered severe mortality from epidemic disease. In 1641, the worst year of the second outbreak, seventy-nine localities in ten provinces were struck."[19] The outbreaks in the 1820s were caused by the first worldwide pandemic of Asiatic cholera.[20]

Suzhou did not escape from the devastating epidemics which ravaged late Ming and Qing China. Records show that the epidemics in the 1580s and the 1640s were especially calamitous. It was said that the epidemic in 1580 caused a high mortality rate. The high death rate was caused not only by the epidemic but many also died of starvation. It was said to be more severe than the one in 1561.[21] The 1641 epidemic was said to have caused the death of approximately seventy percent of those who fell ill, totaling over ten thousand. The magnitude of the disaster was compared to that of the massacre of the Jin soldiers during the Jianyan (1127–31) period in the Southern Song. The following year saw a gradual abatement of the seriousness of the epidemic when over half of the sick were healed.[22] The 1733 epidemic was also said to have caused widespread mortality.

The identification of the particular epidemics is especially difficult mainly because the sources do not provide enough description of the symptoms. The entries are often only listed as *yi* (pestilence) or *dayi* (great pestilence). The 1641 epidemic is identified as *yili* which probably was a kind of gastro-intestinal disease. However it is also possible that the epidemic in different regions involved more than one kind of disease. The epidemic was spread over large portions of the country, preceded by two years of drought. Zhejiang physician Zhao Qingchu in his *Cuncunzhai yihua gao* (Draft of Medical Words from the Cuncun Studio) mentioned the epidemic as *gedawen* and *yangmaowen*, and death came swiftly. Within eight or nine months the death toll reached several million.[23] The 1820s epidemic of Asiatic cholera was recorded by Suzhou physician Lu Maoxiu who commented that the symptoms were vomiting, abdominal pain, and severe diarrhea which depletes the patient who dies.[24]

This lack of more detailed description of epidemic diseases by the compilers of the local gazetteers and writers of dynastic histories is reflective of the indifference towards the medical aspect of the epidemics. These disasters, regardless of their particular characteristics, were considered less as medical phenomena that required medical attention but rather as problems of a political and administrative nature for the government which must deal with the provision of medical care and relief as a measure of benevolence as well as to maintain order in society.

As the representative of the imperial throne at the local level, the magistrate thus shouldered the dual responsibility of representing the benevolence of the throne to the people, as well as maintaining social order for the imperial government. The fulfillment of this duty of the magistrate was the provision of care during times of disasters. Most often the magistrates would set up a bureau and distribute medicine (*sheju shiyao*). Thus in the 1641 epidemic the magistrate of Wuxian, Niu Ruolin, distributed medicine and also set up a bureau, hiring physicians to treat the sick. *Tuiguan* Ni Changyu joined with him to tend to the task of gathering and burying the bodies left in the open. Niu Ruolin again set up a bureau and distributed medicine in the following year when the region was again struck by an epidemic. This time, however, half of the people were cured and it was obviously not as disastrous as the previous year, although we have little clue as to the nature of the illnesses. Another recorded governmental intervention in times of epidemics was in 1719 when Li Xu reported to the Kangxi (1662–1722) emperor that local officials in Suzhou were setting up pharmacies and selecting physicians to tend to the sick in response to an outbreak of epidemic diseases among the people.[25] During the Qianlong reign (1736–95) in the spring of 1756 Suzhou was visited by a widespread epidemic preceded by famine the previous year. Magistrate Zhao You distributed medicine and recruited twenty-five famous physicians and set up a bureau at the Yuanmiao *guan* (Yuanmiao temple) to treat patients in turns. Many were said to have been saved and by summer the epidemic gradually abated but the mortality rate was still high.[26]

Physicians therefore worked with the magistrates in the treatment of patients during times of epidemics. Huang Liuhong comments that "Medical practitioners in the locality should be requested to attend to the sick refugees by turns, free of charge. Medical supplies used should be reimbursed by the government when the practitioners present their bills. Those who have saved many lives are given commendatory tablets as encouragement."[27] The participation in the relief efforts and the provision of medical services to the sick free of charge can be considered as part of the expression of the moral obligation of the medical profession. In recognition of their services they were not only remunerated for the medicine that they have provided, but recognition also came in the form of tablets extolling their good deeds.

By participating in government-sponsored relief efforts, the physicians also could enhance their standing in society and legitimize their profession. Work in the relief efforts often led to fame. For example in 1756 Zheng Jian, who came from a family of physicians, participated in the relief efforts of magistrate Zhao You and, because he was able to cure many people, his reputation in medicine spread. Physicians who were already well-known for their medical abilities still participated in the relief efforts. For example both Ye Gui and Xue Xue took turns with other physicians to treat the sick during the epidemics in the Qianlong period. For the physicians, this association with the governmental efforts was their symbolic expression of their benevolence as well as a legitimization of their professional abilities.

Epidemics were often related to other types of natural disasters, such as flood and drought, that led to food shortages and a breakdown in sanitation. Records often show a series of natural calamities that led to the outbreak of the epidemics. The epidemic in 1580 was preceded by torrential rains that caused floods; and similarly in 1588, the epidemic was preceded by unrelenting rains that flooded the fields and destroyed the crops. The 1641 epidemic, which claimed a seventy percent mortality rate of those affected followed several months of drought and locust infestations. The result was ensuing famine and the soaring of the price of rice.[28]

To what extent the medications used at the time effective in fighting the epidemic diseases is still unclear. In our discussion on the development and maturation of the *wenbing* (heat factor) theory in Chapter Three, it is clear that physicians such as Wu Youxing developed new ideas concerning the nature and transmission of communicable diseases. The effort to impose a new framework upon epidemic diseases also represented the increasing demands on specialization within the medical profession. Debates over the methods of the Heat Factor school illustrates the tensions among the different practitioners of medicine. Physicians were not, however, relied upon for the maintenance of social order. It was the officials who were responsible for the maintenance of the well-being of the people and the society.

Table 4 Records of Epidemics in Suzhou during the Ming and Qing

Year	Description
1454	dayi* many died
1492	dayi
1545	dayi
1561	dayi
1580	flood,yi, many died, worse than 1561
1588	flood, dayi
1641	yili**, 70% died
1642	dayi
1680 summer	dayi
1709	yiqi, provision of medicine
1733	yili, many dead
1746	dayi (Gu Yue tongshantang)
1756	dayi (Zhao You provided medicine)
1786	dayi
1821	dayi
1891	yizheng***, vomiting, diarrhea,

* *dayi* great pestilence
** *yili* pestilence
*** *yizheng* pestilence

Sources: MGWXZ, CZWXZ, SZFZ, WMBZ, JSYR

Benevolent Medicine in Suzhou

The Qing legal codes included the provision of relief for the poor and destitute, the responsibility for which rested mainly upon the local magistrates[29]:

> All poor destitute widowers and widows, the fatherless and children, the helpless and the infirm, shall receive sufficient maintenance and protection from the magistrates of their native city or district, wherever they have neither relations nor connections upon whom they can depend for support. Any magistrate refusing such maintenance and protection, shall be punished with 60 blows.
>
> Also when any such persons are maintained and protected by government, the superintending magistrate and his subordinates, if failing to afford them the legal allowance of food and raiment, shall be punished in proportion to the amount of the deficiency, according to the law against an embezzlement of government stores.

In practice, however, there was no specific allocation of funds for the setting up of charitable associations, and it was up to the individual magistrates to initiate their setup.

Many local charitable associations originated with the Qing government's major agencies for the welfare of the less fortunate, these consisted of the *yangjiyuan*, the *pujitang.*, and the *yuyingtang.* The local gazetteers in Suzhou listed numerous philanthropic associations and welfare agencies that were designed to serve the unfortunate and destitute. Some of these did take in people who were sick and offered medical care to those who could not afford to see a physician. In this sense they were similar to the hospitals in the West in this period of time, which also mainly served the poor and those who could not afford their own physicians. They were also similar in that these institutions were seen as charitable organizations rather than institutions of medical care. The state was interested in the provision of medical care not only in extraordinary times such as epidemics, but also in ordinary times as welfare for the poor. The medicine that the state patronized was the learned tradition, and physicians were chosen according to the non-institutional criteria that were set up.

The provision of medical welfare for the people consisted of both state-sponsored institutions and private ones. The most prevalent state-sponsored ones included the *huimin yaoju* (Pharmacy for the Benefit of the People) and the *pujitang* (Charitable Hall). In looking at the provision of welfare in Suzhou, we find that the state maintained an overwhelming presence in its moral and symbolic control while there was the emergence of a "public sphere" in which the elite sponored and operated many of the charitable institutions. Yet, even these elite sponsored institutions came under the paternalistic moral influence of the state.

The tradition of the provision of medicine and medical care in Suzhou parallels the national trend. The first *Taiping huimin yaoju* in Suzhou was set up in 1195, during the Southern Song dynasty to distribute medicine.[30] It was continued during the Yuan dynasty and the Yuan government was particularly concerned with matters of health. An edict issued during the reign of Dade (1297–1307) called for the setting up of the Pharmacies in the *lu* (circuits) and *fu* (prefectures). The Suzhou pharmacy was rebuilt in 1318.[31] The Hongwu emperor (reign 1368–1398) in the Ming issued decrees in 1370 and also set up a Pharmacy, although not much is known about it. This policy of setting up public pharmacies for the distribution of medicine to the poor was not continued into the Qing and the sources do not list any *huimin yaoju.*

The *huimin yaoju* were government initiated, and it is difficult to discern the extent to which physicians played a role in the administration. The Yuan Pharmacy was staffed by physicians rotating for a year. These government pharmacies undoubtedly assumed their most important role during times of famine and epidemics. The discontinuation in the Qing did not mean that there were no distributions of medicine in times of need. Charitable associations set up by private individuals such as the *yirentang* (1856) and the *huiantang.* (1806) continued in their efforts to provide for the needy.

On the third day of the sixth month of the fifty-fifth year of Kangxi (1716), an auspicious day selected especially for this occasion, Li Xu, the Suzhou *zhizao*[32] (Superintendent of Imperial Silk Manufacturing), Cao Fu[33] and Wu Cunli led the dedication of the plaque with the characters *xiangyanpuji* written by the emperor on it for the *pujitang* (charitable hall) in Suzhou.[34] By bestowing the plaque upon the charitable hall, the emperor strove to portray himself as a benevolent ruler concerned with the plight of the less fortunate. It also emphasized the symbolic power of the emperor over his people and served to extend the influence of the imperial state on local affairs.

This *pujitang* was the *nanpujitang.* (charitable hall for men) located in Changzhou county and was established in 1710 through donations by a group of gentry led by Gu Rulong for the purpose of taking care of the sick and poor. The dedication of the plaque by the emperor was accompanied a grant of funds for the purchase of eight *qing* forty-four *mu* of land. In addition the local gentry also contributed to the purchase of two *qing* sixty *mu* of land. In 1766 there was an addition of 51 sickrooms.[35]

This dedication was significant in two aspects. It underlined the importance of the *pujitang* in Suzhou during this time and was an indicator of strong state interest in the provision of welfare for the people in Suzhou. In Wuxian the *pujitang* was for women. It was set up in 1738 by local gentry Wu Sanfu for the purpose of accommodating sick women and was funded by income from two *qing* of land. Six years later in 1744 it was given twenty-eight *qing* of land the government had confiscated which stabilized the financial condition of the charitable hall. It was destroyed in 1860 by the Taiping armies and rebuilt during the Tongzhi (r. 1862–74) reign by Feng Guifen with the incorporation of the x*ileitang,* which was set up in 1735 for the purpose of burying the poor. This incorporation added the amount of land under the *pujitang's* control with land variously in Wuxian, Changzhou and other counties providing income.

Therefore while the two *pujitang* in Wuxiang and Changzhou were both privately initiated and managed by local gentry, it remained under the moral control of the state and received financial aid in the form of public land. This distinguished it from the public sphere as described by Habermas in which the organizations were formed independent of the state.

Aside from the two *pujitang* for men and women, there were also other charitable associations which provided medical care for needy people. For example in Wuxian the h*uiantang*, y*irentang*, and the w*eiyutang* all provided either medicine or offered medical care. The h*uiantang* was established in 1806 by Xu Xiaobiao. It provided coffins and burial as well as medicine. It was destroyed by fire in 1860 and rebuilt in the late 1860s. The h*uiantang* however did not receive any government allotted land and received land in donations.[36] The y*irentang.*, located in Guangfu *zhen*, was built in 1856 by Feng Guifen because Guangfu was the only place without such an association to help the poor in times of need. It provided coffins and medicine and also set up a *zhongshuju* (tree planting bureau) for financing. Later it received land from the county.[37]

The Suzhou gentry were very much involved in the setting up and maintenance of charitable associations. Although many later did receive land from the county to finance the association, they were initially private initiatives. Suzhou physician Lu Maoxiu also set up a charitable association by the name of *Yongyuan ju* in 1871.[38] It is unclear, however, if the association received money from the state.

Thus even though the state did not initiate charitable associations in late imperial Suzhou, it maintained symbolic influence and control over them through the provision of government land. The management of the associations, however, was almost always left in the hands of the gentry. Many times, however, as in the case of the *yirentang*, Feng Guifeng had strong ties with the government which undoubtedly helped in his obtaining governmental land and sponsorship. Therefore in late imperial times, the government increasingly ceded direct involvement in local health and disaster relief into the hands of the local gentry, while maintaining symbolic moral authority through provision of financial support through the granting of land.

Notes

[1]"*Siqi Tiaoshen Dalun Pian*" in *Huangdi neijing suwen* (The Inner Canon of the Yellow Emperor: Basic Questions) in *Gujin tushu jicheng yibu quanlu* (A Complete Collection of Works Past and Present: Medicine) vol.12 (Hong Kong: Yuguan chubanshe) p.4.

[2] *Zhouli (Rituals of Zhou), Tianguan zhongzai* in *Zhongguo wenhua jinghua quanji: Yixue juan* (Complete Collection of the Essence of Chinese Culture: Medicine) (Beijing: Zhongguo Guoji Guanbo chubanshe, 1992), p. 1.

[3] For more detailed discussion on Tang medical policies see Michihata, Yoshihide 道端良秀. "Tôdai jiin no shaki jigyô: hita yôbyôbô nitsuite," 唐代寺院の社會事業：悲田養病坊に就いて (Social Welfare of the Tang Monasteries-Hospices for the Sick) in *Eizan Gakuhô* 叡山學報 15:18–26.

[4]*Xintangshu* . See also Zheng Qiao. *Tongzhilue.Zhiguan* 6.

[5]*Xintangshu*

[6]According to Zheng Qiao's *Tongzhilue* 14:*Zhiguanlue* 6, the *Guanji fang* (Extensive Relief Prescriptions) was published in 723 and the *Guangli fang* (Extensive Beneficial Prescriptions) was published in 796.

[7] The *huimin yaoju,* however, had its critics. For example Zhou Mi attacked corrupt officials who stole medicine and replaced it with imitations and prepared medicine that went to high officials instead of the needy. *Guixin zashi* in *Jindi mishu.* Shen Gua also criticized the *huimin yaoju* as benefitting the powerful rather than the people.

[8] *Yuanshi*

[9] *Yuanshi*

[10] Angela Leung, "Organized Medicine in Ming-Qing China: State and Private Medical Institutions in the Lower Yangzi Region," in *Late Imperial China* 8.1 (June 1987): 134–166.

[11]William T. Rowe, *Hankow: Conflict and Community in a Chinese City, 1796–1895* (Stanford: Stanford University Press, 1989), p. 99.

[12] Pierre-Etienne Will, *Bureaucracy and Famine in Eighteenth-Century China*, translated from the French by Elborg Forster (Stanford: Stanford University Press, 1990).

[13] Pierre-Etienne Will and R. Bin Wong, *Nourish the People: The State Civilian Granary System in China, 1650–1850 (Michigan: Center for Chinese Studies, University of Michigan, 1991).* especially pp. 497–502.

[14] *Mingshi* (History of Ming), *zhiguan* (Offices), *zhi* 51.

[15] MGWXZ, *gongshu* 2, 29b:24a.

[16] MGWXZ, 29b:6b.

[17] Huang Liu-hung, *A Complete Book Concerning Happiness and Benevolence—A Manual for Local Magistrates in the Seventeenth Century China*, translated by Djang Chu (Tuscon: University Arizona Press, 1984), p. 560.

[18] Helen Dunstan has done extensive research on the first two of these epidemics and her work remains the most comprehensive. Her article "The Late Ming Epidemics: A Preliminary Survey" in *Ch'ing-shih Wen-t'i*, 3.3: 1–59, is based mainly on the local gazetteers and incidental references in historical and literary writings. The Japanese scholar Imura Kôzen has attempted the enormous task of compiling epidemic records from gazetteers and, though still plagued by many problems, remains one of the most comprehensive. Mark Elvin has also dealt with the issue of the late Ming epidemics in *The Pattern of the Chinese Past,* especially pp.310–312.

[19] Mark Elvin, *The Pattern of the Chinese Past*, p. 310.

[20] There were altogether eight worldwide pandemics of Asiatic cholera in the nineteenth and twentieth centuries. The first pandemic from 1817–1823 originated in India and spread by land to China and Ceylon, then by sea to Mauritius, East Africa, the Philippines and Japan. It also spread to Iran, Arabia and Russia. For details see Wesley W. Spink, *Infectious Diseases: Prevention and Treatment in the Nineteenth and Twentieth Centuries* (Minneapolis: University of Minnesota Press, 1978), p. 163.

[21] CZWXZ, *xiangyi*

[22] CZWXZ, *xiangyi*, MGWXZ, *xiangyi*

[23] Zhao Jinchu, *Cuncunzhai yihua yao*, *juan* 2:31. 1883 edition. *Zhenben yishu jicheng* v. 14 (Shanghai: Shanghai Kexue jishu chubanshe, 1986).

[24] Lu Maoxiu, *Shibuzai yishu*, 16:13a.

[25] *Suzhou Zhizao Li Xxu Zouzhe* , p. 69.

[26] MGWXZ, *liezhuan yishu* 75a:38b, also SZFZ, *zaji* 149:7a.

[27] Huang Liu-hung, p. 566.

[28] CZWXZ, *xiangyi*

[29] *Da Qing Luli*, translated by G.T. Staunton, p.93.

[30] GSZ, 22: 33b, also MGWXZ, 29b:22b.

[31] MGWXZ, 29b:24b.

[32] The Qing continued the Ming practice of appointing Superintendents of silk manufacturing in the areas of Jiangning (present day Nanjing), Suzhou, and Hangzhou.

[33] The Cao family had been prominent in political affairs and his father Cao Yin had been the Jiangning and Suzhou *zhizao* with special favor with the Kangxi emperor.

[34] *Suzhou Zhizao Li Xu Zouzhe* (Superintendent of Imperial Silk Manufacturing Li Xu's Memorials to the Throne) (Taibei: Wenhai chubanshe, 1977), p. 197.

[35] SZFZ, p.568.

[36] MGWXZ, 30:11b.

[37] Ibid. 30:11a.

[38] MGWXZ, 30:14a.

CHAPTER SIX

Practicing Medicine: Specialization and the Transmission of Medical Knowledge

MEDICINE is of necessity a practical and a technical profession. The increase in the number of elite physicians in late imperial China provided impetus for the clear articulation of a medical ethic and qualifications of an ideal physician that was cemented through literary networks. However this did not alter the fundamental character of the medical profession as one which possessed specialized knowledge. Even in their attempts to establish legitimacy over the hereditary physicians and in debates over the importance of text over experience, the Confucian physicians did not deny the necessity for technical knowledge. This emphasis on specialized knowledge had been an important component of the classical medical tradition.

This chapter will look at the emergence of the *yi* (physician) as a specialized function and the development of specializations and specialized knowledge in medical practice that separated the layman from the physician. Since there were no formal criteria for licensing and evaluation of physicians, they could practice medicine simply by hanging up a symbolic gourd. Therefore reputation based on efficacy played a major role both in the evaluation and regulation of the practice of medicine.

Yi as A Specialized Profession: Separation of *yi* and *wu*

The late Ming Suzhou physician Wu Youxing recounts the story of a patient in his *Wenyilun* (Treatise on Warm Factor Epidemic Diseases). The patient, a man by the name of Shi Yousheng who made a decent living making divinations (*bu*), became ill with symptoms which on the surface seemed like *yinzheng* (*yin* factor illness). Most physicians consulted concurred that it was an illness of the yin factor, but Wu believed that the symptoms masked the true nature of the illness which he believed to be of a yang nature and prescribed different medication. Shi's wife upon hearing the different diagnoses of both a yin illness and a yang illness was at a loss as to which side to listen to. His brother consulted three physicians in a row who all diagnosed it to be of a yin illness. The patient then told his wife to use divination to determine which diagnosis was correct. The result of the divination was that "To follow the yin will be auspicious, to follow the yang will be unfortunate."[1] Based on the result of the divination and the fact that most physicians believed it to be a yin illness, the patient took the medicine of the other physicians but soon died. Wu Youxing lamented, "Alas! [He has] always used divination as a means of livelihood, in the end it is divination which caused [his] death. This can serve as a warning of shaman and diviners!"[2]

This episode not only shows that divination was quite popular among the people by that fact that Shi Yousheng was able to make a decent living by this trade, but it also indicated the disdain the physicians in general had for those who consulted the supernatural, either soliciting their fortune or seeking treatment of their illnesses. This objection came from two concerns. The first was the different ideological and theoretical foundation for treatment, and the second was a concern either consciously or unconsciously about competition for patients.

Although the use of shamanist methods of healing did not disappear from the medical tradition, even from the elite medical tradition, in the process of the adoption of the Confucian ethics and alliance with the dominant intellectual tradition, the elite tradition found it necessary to distance itself from the folk traditions of healing in which shamanism and divinations played a major role. The attitude of Wu Youxing towards the patient represented a culmination of the process of a long process of separation of the *yi* from the *wu* tradition.

From the literature on the discussions about the history of medicine in China, the roots of the *yi* (physician) in China were often traced back to the *wu* (shaman), who were thought to possess magical powers in their ability to call on supernatural forces. Illness and disease were often thought to be caused by the supernatural and thus prayer was one of the major forms of healing. From the oracle bone inscriptions, there is evidence showing that the *wu* healed with prayers as well as with drugs.[3] The *wu* in Shang (1700–1100 B.C.) China were considered to be the elite who possessed the charisma[4] to establish a special relationship with the divine gods. Shangdi, the supreme being, was amoral but controlled forces of the world and could be influenced through the ancestor gods. Therefore rituals and sacrifices to these gods were a vital part of kingship. The king was the head shaman due to his unique ability to communicate with the gods.

The redefinition of the relationship with the divine by the Zhou (1100–256 B.C.) rulers and the emerging concept of a moral *Tian* (heaven) eroded the political status of the *wu*. Power in the Zhou was no longer obtained through charisma but through moral conduct and political legitimacy was sanctioned by the Mandate of Heaven. The *wu* therefore lost their political importance as a medium between the divine and the people, but they retained the function of healing and of communication with the supernatural world.

Incidences of the activities of the *wu* are evident in historical writings, and it is from the lamentations of the scholars and Confucian physicians on the "superstition" of the common people who used the *wu* to attempt to cure illnesses that we can assume consultation of the *wu* was still widely practiced. It was not only among the common people but can be found among the elite as well. There are many references in the classical sources to the healing function of the *wu*. For example in *Lunyu* (The Analects), it is said that "The southerners have a saying: `A man without persistence cannot become a sorcerer-physician (*wuyi*, shaman-physician). Good."[5] Wang Fu of the Later Han also criticized those who looked to shamans, not physicians, for cure in his *Qianfulun* :

> If one wants to know when a person is going to become ill, [it is by the symptom that] he does not want to eat; if one wants to know when a country is going to perish, [it is by the fact that] it does not covet the virtuous. It is not that the person does not have sumptuous food, but he is ill and cannot eat, thus dying; it is not that the country lacks virtuous people, but it does not use them, thus it perishes quickly. For the ruling of the country to not have true virtuous people, is like curing an illness without a true physician.[6]

The downfall of the political status of the *wu* coincided with the growing separation of its magical healing function from the classical tradition of medicine, which was in its formative stages at this time. The latter incorporated the concepts of the *yin/yang* and five phases into its theoretical framework. The alliance with Confucian ideas of the perfect gentleman was also made, which provided the basis for the formation of an ethics for the practice of medicine by the elite. The healer and the shaman parted company, though not completely, as we shall later see. The functions of healing became more autonomous with the accumulation of knowledge about diseases, the healing power of the myriad natural resources through practical experience ,and the formation of a written tradition in medicine.

Even though the distance between the *yi* and the *wu* widened, the tension between the *yi* and other shamanic forms of healing remained. Physicians since Bian Que have derided patients who refused to accept their treatment but instead resorted to prayers and appealed to the supernatural powers. For example the Jin physician Zhang Congzheng (1156–1228) in his *Rumen shiqin* (Confucians' Duties to Their Parents) tells of an account of a man in his sixties who believed that his ailments were caused by spirits and continuously prayed to ghosts and spirits but to no avail. He was finally cured when Zhang Congzheng prescribed a cooling formula which purged him of the impurities in his body and restored his health.[7]

The physicians in traditional China not only distrusted the shamans, they also criticized the *fangshi* who sought ways of longevity, many through alchemy. As the elite level of the medical tradition moved closer to the classical Confucian tradition, there were efforts to disassociate physicians the healing traditions in Daoism, Buddhism, and other folk traditions. Li Shizhen (1518–1655), the famous Ming pharmacologist who compiled the *Bencao gangmu* (Compendium of *Materia Medica*), attacked the *fangshi* as unworthy of consideration and gave many instances of the harmful, sometimes deadly, effects of engaging in alchemical pursuits.

However, despite the attempts by the elite physicians to distance themselves from the folk healers and their various attempts to discredit the folk traditions of healing, this does not mean that there was a clear line demarcating the division of elite and folk medicine. There was still constant interaction between the two traditions and a fluid relationship.[8] Li Shichen himself, who was called a would-be Confucian by some,[9] and who was particularly impressed with the Song philosopher Zhu Xi, did not reject shamanistic healing and believed in the possession of spirits. It was clear therefore that the elite physicians, though they professed disdain for the folk and religious healers, did not necessarily reject their conceptions of sickness and methods of therapy. In the Imperial Medical Academy, from the Tang onwards till the Ming, *zhuyou* (shamanist healing) was one of the thirteen specializations recognized and an examination subject.

The *wu* tradition of healing was separated from the classical tradition in medicine which was forming at this time and which attempted to establish its monopoly over healing. However the wu never disappeared from the realm of healing and continued to perform important healing and religious functions in the folk tradition.

Yi as a Specialized Function

The image of the Chinese scholar as an amateur ideal with a disdain for technical knowledge and specialization has been expounded by scholars who considered that the gentry elite in late imperial China was one immersed in the ideal of the perfect Confucian, indulging in non-technical, non-specialized studies. They did not pursue the useful, but rather the artistic. Thus Levenson comments that "Artistic style and a cultivated knowledge of the approved canon of ancient works, the `sweetness and light' of a classical love of letters—these, not specialized, `useful' technical training, were the tools of intellectual expression and the keys to social power.[10] He concludes, "The Ming style was the amateur style; Ming culture was the apotheosis of the amateur."[11] Fei Xiaotong considered the Chinese gentry as "a class without technical knowledge. They monopolized authority based on the wisdom of the past, spent time on literature, and tried to express themselves through art."[12]

This picture of the ideal amateur Confucian has been successfully challenged by recent scholarship and the recognition of a process by the Qing scholars towards academic professionalization.[13] Late imperial Jiangnan saw an influx of Confucian scholars into the group of physicians. These physicians had chosen medicine as a career not just for its linkage with the classical tradition, but their writings also show an understanding of the importance of specialized knowledge in medicine, and the recognition of medicine as a specialized function based on a tradition of specialized medical knowledge.

The process by which the *yi* (physician) became a specialized group in healing based on expert knowledge was probably accomplished during the Chunqiu (Spring and Autumn 722–481 B.C.) and Zhanguo (Warring States 403–222 B.C.) periods. This separation of the physician and the shaman is apparent in the account of Qin Yueren in *Shiji* (Records of History), written by the Han (206 B.C. to 220 A.D.) historian Sima Qian (145–87 B.C.?) in which one of the six incurable diseases mentioned was the belief in *wu* rather than in *yi*.[14] Thus the line between the two was already drawn sharply. It was also an indication of competition between the two in terms of patients. Success in the latter was important in that the physician, if he was to survive as a profession of healing, needed to establish his legitimacy. This attack on the people's belief in shamans and use of them in the treatment of illness is evidence that many people still sought the shaman for cures. To counter the power of the shamans, the physicians thus had to legitimize their own forms of healing. This was done by the formulation of a medical tradition through the accumulation of knowledge and experience, leading to knowledge of specializations within the field, and later utilization of the dominant Confucian tradition to bolster its claims of moral legitimacy.

This break between the functions of the shaman and the physician is also expressed in the medical classic *Huangdi neijing* (The Inner Canon of the Yellow Emperor). For example it states that, "For those who believe in spirits and gods, [one cannot] discuss with them the ultimate virtues; for those who dislike [the use of] needles and stone needles, [one cannot] discuss with them the utmost skills [of medicine]."[15] Thus the authors of the period of the *Huangdi neijing* already had distinguished between those who believed in the supernatural and those who utilized the medical knowledge of acupuncture. It also served to show that by that time, there was already the beginning of the formation of specializations in medicine, in particular the use of sharpened stones and needles as healing tools.

In the process of separating from the magical, the *yi* began to develop specialization within the field and criteria of evaluation within their own ranks. The *Zhouli* (Rituals of Zhou)[16] records an emerging system of medical care in which there was not only the ranking of physicians and specification of duties, but also the beginnings of specialization in the practice of medicine. The appearance of ranking for the physicians and the resultant hierarchy indicated not only the growth of a group of individuals who performed healing functions but, more importantly, it was the beginnings of the construction of a boundary for the physicians. It was a boundary both of exclusion and inclusion. It excluded those who did not meet the criteria and included those deemed qualified.

There were altogether five categories of specialization of physicians mentioned in the Rituals of Zhou: the *yishi* (general physician), *shiyi* (physician of diet), *jiyi* (physician of illness), *yangyi* (physician of wounds and skin infection), *shouyi* (physician of animals).[17] Each group was then divided into different ranks. The *yishi* (general physicians), who were at the top of the hierarchy of these five groups of physicians, were ranked as *shangshi*, *xiashi*, *fu*, *shi*, and *tu*.[18] Their function was to be in charge of the administrative duties of health and medicine, the gathering of medicinal drugs, and the supervision and evaluation of the other groups of physicians.

Elite medicine traces its lineage back to the legendary three emperors: Huangdi (Yellow Emperor),[19] Shennong (Divine Farmer), and Fuxi (Ox-tamer). Fuxi is credited with inventing the use of fire and lessening instances of illness with cooked food, Shennong is thought to have laid the basis of pharmaceutical knowledge with his experiments with the various herbals. Huangdi is credited with the development of a set of medical theory which laid the basis for the theoretical foundation of traditional Chinese medicine.

The oldest source of extant medical writings available today are the manuscripts excavated from Mawangdui site in the 1970s near Changsha in Hunan province. It is speculated that the materials there were dated at around the end of the third century B.C. or second century B.C. The medical texts found not only contained shamanistic healing but also showed the beginnings of a systematic attempt at the classification of medical knowledge using the yin-yang idea of polarity and the concepts of the five evolutionary phases (*wuxing*).

The philosophical flourishing which occurred in the later Zhou period found expression not only in the so-called hundred different schools of thought but also helped the formulation of a medical tradition that was to dominate medical theory and therapy in the classical medical tradition for the next two thousand years. Two works that were later canonized were the *Huangdi neijing* and the *Shennong bencaojing*. Physicians and students of medicine were expected to be familiar with the ancient medical classics attributed to the legendary sovereigns. The purpose was not only to be familiar with the theoretical foundations but also a form of legitimacy in claiming to be the intellectual descendent of the ancients.

The most authoritative ancient medical classic is the *Huangdi neijing* (Inner Canon of the Yellow Emperor). Although it is attributed to the legendary sovereign Huangdi, it probably was compiled over a period of a century and put together some time in the first century B.C.. However the two extant parts which make up the *Neijing*, the *Suwen* (Basic Questions) and the *Lingsu* (Divine Pivot), probably did not exist in their present form until the eighth century. The *Huangdi bashiyi Nanjing* (Canon of Eighty-one Problems of the Yellow Emperor) though sometimes attributed to Qin Yueren, was probably compiled during the second century A.D.. Although it purports to explore the difficulties in the *Neijing*, indications are that it probably came from a separate medical tradition.

It was some time during the third or fourth century B.C. that the dualistic and complementary *yin* and *yang*, and the *wuxing* (five evolutionary phases) concepts were developed to regulate natural phenomena. They were incorporated into the medical tradition and became the basis for the development of medical theories of diagnosis and therapy. The excavated materials at the Mawangdui showed rudimentary utilization whereas in the *Huangdi neijing* we find a more elaborate use of the system of correspondences. However in the canonized medical work, the *Shennong Bencaojing*, we find relatively little use of the system. It was the prince of Huainan, Liu An (died 122 B.C.) of the Han who made the connection between the legendary Shennong and the beginnings of pharmaceutics in the work *Huainanzi* (Writings of the Prince of Huainan). The *Shennong Bencaojing* (Divine Husbandman's Materia Medica) was probably compiled some time during the second century A.D.

Conceptions of the social order and the hierarchical relationships between the ruler and the ruled often find expression in medical terms. The analogy between sickness and the disruption of social order is a recurring theme not only in medical literature but also in Confucian writings. The *Huangdi neijing* proclaims, "The sage does not cure those who are already ill, but those who are not yet ill. They do not order the state when there is trouble, but order the state before trouble begins."[20] Thus in the *Neijing* drugs are divided into categories of *jun* (ruler), *chen* (minister), *zuo* (assistant), *shi* (aide). The *jun* are those that are effective in the curing of the illness, reflecting not only the hierarchical relationship of ruler and officials, but also the Confucian concern of the ruler and his duty in the maintenance of social order.

We find a different kind of concern and categorization of drugs in the *Shennong bencaojing*. Drugs are also categorized according to their effectiveness in treatment and divided into a similar scheme to that of the Neijing. However the best drugs, the *jun*, are those that are not used for curing diseases but rather for longevity and thus contains no `poison'. The least desirable were those that combated acute diseases. It thus reflected a more Daoist concern of the ruler as a person who maintained harmony rather than order. This Daoist tradition is even more pronounced later in Tao Hongjing's (456–536) pharmaceutical works. Daoist concern for longevity and the development of alchemical techniques have made an impression in the development of the pharmaceutical tradition in China.

It was thus various social forces and intellectual impulses that contributed to the formation of a written medical tradition in China. Later foreign influences such as Buddhism and medical innovations from India were also to leave marks upon the evolving medical tradition. However the development of this literate tradition also meant that part of the medical knowledge became restricted to the literate sector of society. The specialized function of the *yi* came to rest upon familiarity with written texts.

Criteria of Assessment: Reputation

The main criteria for the maintenance of membership within the group was based upon the efficacy of their treatments. They were judged based on their rates of success and failure in treating patients. Therefore the earliest evaluation system found in the Book of Rites stated that those who cured ten out of ten (100% rate of cure) of the patients were considered the best, those who failed one in ten were the next best (90% rate of cure), then those who failed twice (80% rate of cure), then three times (70% rate of cure). Finally those who failed four times (60% rate of cure) were considered inferior.[21] This emphasis on the efficacy of treatments was to remain a major criterion of judgment in traditional Chinese medicine. Even with the increasing alliance with the Confucian tradition and the formulation of a medical ethic based on Confucian morality, efficacy continued to play an important role in the validation of the status of a physician. This became especially important in a society in which official sanction and licensing of the medical profession did not develop.[22] Reputations of physicians thus became one of the most important criteria for the judgment of a physician's competence, and reputation was based upon the efficacy of their treatments. Sivin also believes that it is efficacy which explains why elite physicians adopted ritual therapies and folk remedies in their treatments at times. Elite physicians chose symbolic therapies which were meaningful to their patients. [23]

Some physicians at times solicited written testimonies (essays, letters, or poems) attesting to the effective treatments from their high-status patients, something akin to a letter of recommendation. Ming scholar Zhang Chai became afflicted with what physicians called *xuanyong* (carbuncle of the perineum) and *nangyong* (abscess of scrotum). As his condition worsened his friends urged him to consult the then famous *yangke* (wounds/skin infection) physician Qiao Zongfu, whose father Qiao Xinyu was also famous in *yangke*. However Zhang was afraid that the treatment would be extremely painful and deferred. Qiao Zongfu then showed Zhang an essay written by his former patient Gao Zhongxian attesting not only to the efficacy of his treatments, but also used the analogy of a gentleman (*junzi*) eliminating petty people (*xiaoren*) to describe Qiao's techniques. Zhang acquiesced after reading the essay. Qiao's treatment was successful at the second try and the whole treatment took about one hundred days. After Zhang was cured, Qiao requested an essay similar to that which was given to him by Gao Zhongxian.[24]

Thus apparently physicians used these "letters of recommendation" to solicit patients and as a testimony of the effectiveness of their treatments. Without formal licensing, these letters and essays served as evidence of their competence as a physician. These written testimonies from literati were especially useful in soliciting patients from the elite and gave them a special standing among the practicing physicians. These letters were written in the language of Confucian rhetoric and therefore, by endorsing the technique and specialized knowledge of the physician, they had still to be placed within the Confucian framework of ideology.

Physicians were also apparently aggressive in soliciting clients as evidenced by the fact that when Zhang initially hesitated in seeking treatment from Qiao, it was the latter who took the initiative to show him the essay from Gao to convince him of his competence. These essays/letters evidently were useful in enhancing the reputation of the physicians. On the other hand the literati were also concerned with their reputations. Zhang recounts an episode in which a Mr. Zhu, delighted with the *fangshiyi* (Daoist physician) who cured his foot ailment, wrote a poem for him. However after a month the ailment recurred and was more severe. He ardently searched for the Daoist physician to retrieve his poem, but the latter had already gone far away. Zhang himself also experienced a relapse of his ailment within five years and was bedridden for almost three years. Although Qiao Zhongfu was nearby and Zhang could have retrieved his essay, he did not do so, reasoning that even if he did get it back from Qiao, it had already been much passed around and that taking it back would not make much difference.[25]

The spread of reputation could be obtained not only though the word of mouth but also through published materials. Late imperial Jiangnan also witnessed a surge in the publication of medical treatises such as case books, collectanea, medical discourses, and primers for the common people (see Chapter 3). The network formed by these physicians served as an arena for advertising their medical knowledge. Through the case books, the physicians were also able to attest to the efficacy of their treatments and thus expand their reputation.

It is clear, however, that the written materials were useful in the recruitment of patients from the gentry families. It was also this type of patient who was desirable because of the potential for high rewards and the opportunity for establishing a relationship with a gentry family. Thus publication became also a means of establishing one's credentials.

Specialization in medical practice

The development of specialized knowledge within the field necessitated a process of learning and a network of patronage for the transmission of this knowledge, thus separating the laymen from the specialist. This process of the transmission of medical knowledge, to be discussed in more detail in the following section, was achieved mainly through apprenticeship and through book-learning.

The four categories of medicine mentioned above, which appeared in the *Zhouli* (Rituals of Zhou) represented the earliest forms of specialization in medicine with each type of physician responsible for not just different symptoms, but for possessing special medical knowledge to treat the different ailments for men and for animals.

The division of special functions in medicine continued in the Sui and Tang periods with the introduction of *anmo boshi* (learned masseur)and *zhoujin boshi* (learned incantor). The Tang saw the addition of the division of *zhenke* (acupuncture) in its Imperial Medical Academy. The formal division of medicine into specialized fields began in the Sung when there were a total of thirteen divisions set up.[26] This set of divisions was continued on into the Ming and Qing dynasties with some modifications. The Ming continued with the thirteen divisions while the Qing began with eleven but eventually modified them into nine. During the Daoguang period (1821–50) *zhenjiuke* (acupuncture and moxibustion) was abolished and later during the Guangxu reign (1875–1908) things were further condensed into five categories: 1. *dafangmai* (adult); 2. *xiaofangmai* (pediatrics); 3. *waike* (external injuries); 4. *yanke* (eye); 5. *kouchike* (mouth and teeth).

Categorization into specializations in the Imperial Medical Academy was a reflection of the development of medicine in general and the accumulation of knowledge concerning the difference in illnesses and diseases. This was reflected in the practice of medicine in the local areas.

In Suzhou, among the physicians who were active in medicine, many were commented upon as being competent in different specialized fields. There was a general recognition among physicians at the time of the importance of specialized knowledge and that different illnesses should be treated by physicians who were knowledgeable in that particular field. Thus Wujiang physician Xu Dachun in his commentary on Ye Gui's *Linzheng zhinan yian* (Collection of Medical Cases for A Guide to Diagnosis) concurred with the commentary on a case which stated that Ye was not a *yangyi* (wounds and skin infection physician). He commented that[27]:

> For the treatment of illnesses there must be a specialist. All kinds of *wan* (pills), *san* (power) and other external methods of healing, once there is unpreparedness, then it cannot establish success in healing. Although the principle is the same yet there are different methods for each. If [one desires] to cure external illnesses, [one] must possess another kind of skill.

In another place he also mentioned the presence of specialist in eye diseases. For those who wished to study the subject more there were specialized works available.[28]

There were many physicians in Suzhou who specialized in wounds and skin infection (*yangke*) and among them the most famous and the most influential was Wang Weide.[29] The exact dates for him are uncertain but he was active during the early Qing period and his work, *Waike zhengzhi quanshengji* (Complete Works for the Diagnosis and Treatment of External Injuries), was published in the fifth year of the Qianlong reign (1740) at an age of seventy-two. He was also skilled in divination and has left behind a work named *Bushi zhengzong* (The Orthodox Teachings of Divination).

Wang came from a family of physicians. Family tradition in medicine began with his great-grandfather Wang Ruogu who was a famous physician in external injuries. Although Wang Weide's father and grandfather apparently also practiced medicine, they do not appear in the sources, and it seems that it was Wang Weide who was more successful in taking up his great grandfather's trade.[30] Wang Ruogu wrote down the formulae which he had found to be effective, and these were passed down from generation to generation, establishing the family tradition of practice in medicine with a specialty in external injuries. Wang Weide's *Waike zhengzhi quanshengji* was based upon his great-grandfather's work. In his preface he explained the reason for publishing his great-grandfather's work supplemented with his own cases was that he believed in this way, many more people could be saved by his methods. Otherwise his practice was only limited to the geographical area of his own village and he could not extend his help to those in other areas. He heard of many people who died needlessly. Therefore he said, "[I] purposely used the secrets passed down by my forefathers, my own cases, and the formula which immediately cures the illness when it is taken, and the methods of refined making of medication. [All are] revealed without any concealment. All are contained in this collection."[31] Wang Weide was said to have regretted very much that he lived in a far away area and could not travel throughout the region. When he heard that someone had died, he always felt extremely saddened.[32] This story, whether true or not, together with his pronouncement of his intentions for publishing his book, served to establish him not only as a skilled physician in external injuries, but also conformed him to the conception of an ideal physician who possessed great compassion for the suffering. It also served to reiterate the importance of benevolence in the judgment of a physician.

Wang Weide therefore did not want to keep the successful treatment methods as *mifang* (secret formula) even though this was a prevalent practice among hereditary physicians at the time. Yet his publication of the work and his claims for his compassion for the sick who cannot benefit from his medical skills elevates his status from that of the common hereditary physician with medical expertise, to one who also possessed the moral virtues of a Confucian. Wang Weide therefore was a physician with the technical skills as well as the moral virtues and worthy to be included among the ranks of physicians in the official and local sources.

In his work, Wang Weide emphasized the importance of distinguishing between the yin and yang of the external ulcers and abscesses. For example a red abscess was considered to be evidence of *yangshi* (congestion of the *yang*) whereas a white abscess indicated *yinxu* (depletion of the yin). His motto for the treatment of all kinds of external ulcers and abscesses was "*yi xiao wei gui, yi tuo wei wei*" (to dissipate as prized, to distend as dread).

Surgical methods, which had been advocated by several physicians in the Ming and apparently widely used by many physicians, suffered a decline during the Qing. This can partly be attributed to the influence of Wang who was adamant in his opposition to the use of surgical methods. Wang was highly critical of those physicians who used surgical methods to cure abscesses or tumors. Thus he criticized Ming physician Chen Shigong (1555–1636)[33] for the latter's advocating of the use of surgery. The use of surgery to treat various ailments had been advocated not only by Chen Shigong but was prevalent among physicians during the Ming. For example Shen Douyuan was fascinated with the surgical procedures allegedly carried out by Hua Tuo and expressed regret that Hua's knowledge was not passed on. His work *Waike qixuan* (Revelation of the Mystery of External Illnesses) discussed many surgical procedures. Together with his contemporary Fu Yunke, a specialist in the eye, he pointed out the importance of boiling the instruments for the purpose of sterilization. Similarly, Wang Kentang (1549–1613), the Ming scholar who retreated from an official career and took up the study of medicine, also described surgical procedures in his work *Waike zhunsheng* (Standards for External Illnesses).

Wang Weide's work during the Qing was widely circulated and he did not mind the work being reprinted. Thus after its first printing in 1740 until 1956, it was reprinted approximately sixty times and during the reign of the Guangxu emperor (1875–1908) alone it was published seventeen times.[34] Many later physicians were influenced by his arguments and took stands against the use of surgery. For this, Wang has been criticized by contemporary scholars for hindering the development of surgery in China and blamed for its decline.[35]

Qing Suzhou physician Yu Mingjian came from a family of five generations of physicians and was a descendant of Yu Shiyue. It was said that when he was over thirty he met a person named Chen from Zhejiang province who gave him a book on acupuncture and also transmitted to him the methods of acupuncture. From then on he specialized in acupuncture and became as famous as Ye Gui and Xue Xue. This family tradition was carried on by his grandson Renhua.[36] Thus it was clear that Yu Mingjian was a physician who was active in Suzhou and famous for his skills in acupuncture. Nevertheless the local gazetteer found it necessary to also mention that he was a person of humble, amiable, upright, and respectful disposition, and was one who never cared for compensation for his services,[37] thus cloaking him in the ideal Confucian physician image of righteousness and benevolence.

Acupuncture had traditionally been a major method of curing illnesses by folk physicians, especially those itinerant healers who traveled from place to place. Their success in making a livelihood depended upon the efficacy of their treatments and since they did not stay in one place long, results needed to be speedy. Thus the popularity of acupuncture and moxibustion among the folk healers. In the local areas, both the elite physicians and the folk physicians, especially the *lingyi* (itinerant physician), practiced acupuncture. Zhao Xuemin (1720–1805) ， in his work *Chuanya neipian* (The Principle Book of Quackery) on the *lingyi* had commented that:

> Carrying a satchel and practicing medicine, travelling around the four corners, is popularly called. This method began with Bian Que, and Hua Tuo followed him, thus the various methods which they pass on, is slightly different from *guoyi* (national physicians).[38] In the treatment of the external [they] mainly used needles to pierce (acupuncture) and steaming to cauterize (moxibustion), in the treatment of the internal [they] mainly used medicines of a *ding*[39] *chuan*[40] nature to restrain and intercept, [it is to] obtain speedy effective results, not for the consideration of the perfect.[41]

Zhao Xuemin's work on itinerant physicians represented an effort on the part of an elite physician to incorporate some of the folk traditions. Although he does not escape using his moral judgments on some of their practices, it is nevertheless an important source on the folk traditions in late imperial China.

Acupuncture had been popular during the Ming dynasty and flourished among the general population. There were also several works written on acupuncture such as Gao Wu's *Zhenjiu juying* (A Synthetical Book of Acupuncture and Moxibustion) published in 1529, and Yang Jizhou's (1522–1620) *Zhenjiu dacheng* (A Comprehensive Collection in Acupuncture and Moxibustion), published in 1601. The former book introduced previous works on acupuncture, discussed the theoretical issues in acupuncture and moxibustion and also practical issues of methods, and finally included songs and poems on acupuncture for easy memorization. Yang's collection was also very comprehensive in its scope and similarly included songs and poems for easy study and memorization. This effort in popularization continued in the Qing dynasty with Wang Ang's *Jingluo gejue* (Secret Song for Meridans) and *Jingluo xuedao ge* (Songs for Meridans and Points).

Xu Dachun was one who believed in the importance of acupuncture. Yet in his view his contemporaries had lost the true transmission of the art of needling and moxa. He lamented not only its lack of prestige but also the deterioration in the skills of the physicians.[42] He said,

> In their detailed discussion of the viscera and of the bowels, of the conduits and their insertion points, and of illness, the Ling [shu] and the Su [wen] refer to prescriptions and drugs only two or three times out of ten,. That shows how much [the people] in high antiquity valued the method of needling. However, learning the doctrine of needling is difficult, while it is easy [to use] prescriptions and drugs. Also, patients enjoy taking drugs, but they suffer from the needles. Hence, in later times the [use of] prescriptions and drugs flourished widely while no one spoke of the method of needling anymore. Today, the application of the needles is marked by ten obvious losses, and that does not even include all the subtleties [that have been forgotten since antiquity].[43]

He then proceeded to discuss the ten losses and finally lamented:

> Today's physicians insert their needles at liberty and do not care about any schema. And even if they were to employ needling methods like the ancients, they would be unable to concentrate their thoughts, and they would not even reach the trigger. Most likely, they would not achieve any good result. How much more is this true, though, for those who turn their backs on the ancient methods![44]

Acupuncture had always been one of the specialties included in the Imperial Medical Academy and was considered part of the necessary curriculum in the Academy. The government also sponsored the study and practice of acupuncture and in 1443 the Ming emperor commissioned the making of a new *zhenjiu tongren* (bronze model for acupuncture) based upon the Song model which came to be known as the *Zhengtong zhenjiu tongren*. A bronze model was also made during the Qing dynasty. The Qianlong emperor (r.1736–95) commissioned physicians Wu Qian and others of the Imperial Medical Academy to compile a collection of medical works. The resultant work, the *Yizong jinjian* (The Golden Mirror of the Orthodox Line of Physicians) still contained works on acupuncture and moxibustion. But in the second year of the Daoguang emperor (r.1821–50), *zhenjiu* was ordered to be abolished in the Imperial Medical Academy: "In the second year of the Daoguang emperor, an imperial order was respectfully received: The method of acupuncture and moxibustion has already been in existence for some time, however using needles to pierce and heat to moxa, is nonetheless not suitable for the serving of the emperor, [thus] the subject of acupuncture and moxibustion in the Imperial Medical Academy is ordered to cease permanently." [45]

It seems that the order to abolish acupuncture was aimed at the Imperial Medical Academy because it was deemed an unsuitable method of treatment for the imperial household, especially the emperor. This is in line with the trend of emphasizing the use of *tangyao* (draught medicine) and a distrust of other forms of medicine and treatments. The official abolition of acupuncture and moxibustion also did not seem to have lowered the position of acupuncture among the physicians, although it did affect the development of this method among the physicians in general. Many Confucian physicians thus considered it unworthy of their study and use.

Transmission of medical knowledge

Medical knowledge was transmitted through both the oral and the literate tradition. Bian Que, the famous physician around fifth century B.C., received the transmission of medical knowledge from Chang Sang Jun. The process involved not only the confirmation of the worthiness of Bian Que to receive the knowledge but also shamanistic and religious ceremonies. The process of medical training for the physician Chunyu Yi involved three stages: oral transmission, confirmation of his ability, and study of ancient texts and practice. [46]

The Confucian physicians often emphasized textual transmission while the hereditary physicians such as Ye Gui placed more emphasis upon the practical experience and personal transmissions. This led to tensions between the two groups and found expression in debates over the interpretation of the ancient classic *Liji* (Book of Rites) which we have discussed.

In their formation of an identity as a group and their attempt to establish a viable tradition, the Suzhou physicians utilized stories and anecdotes to trace their intellectual lineage. The following incident recorded by Yang Xunji in *Sutan* (Conversations on Suzhou) serves to illustrate an attempt to establish the intellectual lineage of Suzhou physicians:

> Nowadays physicians in the Wuzhong area are praised all under heaven. There is a reason for this. At the beginning, Dai Yuanli[47] of Jinhua studied under Zhu Yanxiu[48] and learned his methods entirely. [He] came to the Wu area as a hamlet. People from Wu who consulted him with their illnesses, for every formula written there was a charge of five *liang*. Wang Zhongguang was a Confucian, and did not yet know about medicine. He admired [Dai] and came to pay a visit. He inquired about the way of learning medicine. Yuanli said, "Study the Suwen thoroughly." Zhongguang returned and studied it for three years. Yuanli then came to see Zhongguang again, and was greatly startled after discussion, believing that he himself was not as good, and was afraid that he [Zhongguang] would ruin his practice. Therefore he consolidated the relationship by visiting and paying respects to his mother. At the time although Zhongguang received the teachings from books, he still could not yet put it into practice. Yuanli had ten juan of Yanxiu's medical cases which he kept secretly and refused to teach Zhongguang. Zhongguang privately watched and knew where he hid it. He waited until Yuanli went out and directly took it and returned. Yuanli returned and [realized] he had lost the medical cases and was very repentant... Therefore the fame of Zhongguang spread to all of Suzhou, and that was how physicians in Suzhou began to flourish.[49]

The story in this passage is one that is often told amongst scholars and physicians to trace the beginning of Suzhou as a leading center of medical activities. The line of transmission for Suzhou physicians was thus traced back to Yuan physician Zhu Zhenheng, who was considered as one of the *sidajia* (four great schools).[50] Because he was a famous physician with strong Confucian ties, the tracing of the genealogy of Suzhou physicians back to Zhu Zhenheng endowed them with a sense of legitimacy.

The dispute of the two physicians over the collection of Zhu Yanxiu's medical cases serves to bring out the importance of practical experience in medicine. It also emphasized the transmission of medical knowledge through experience as well as the study of the classics. The *yian* (medical cases) collections throughout the ages were considered an important aspect in the study of medicine. Thus Xu Dachun in his commentary on Ye Gui's *Linzheng zhinan ian* (Medical Cases for Clinical Practice) faults him for collecting too many similar cases and emphasizes that the case histories should select major illnesses and those which others could not cure, so as to set up the standards and to stimulate intellectual thinking and become the rules for followers.[51]

The rivalry between Dai Yuanli and Wang Zongguang and the secrecy regarding methods and formulae were typical of medical practice in late imperial China. One of the most famous feuds between physicians was said to have been between Xue Xue and Ye Gui. Each was said to have been able to cure patients who the other was unable to help.[52]

Effective cures were often jealously guarded to be passed down from generation to generation. The monopoly of a cure would ensure the availability of patients and thus an income. This was often to be found within the families of hereditary physicians when they had established their reputations for a certain specialty. This kind of transmission undoubtedly posed a threat to the scholars turned physicians who did not possess this type of monopoly on cures. Therefore it is not surprising that many Confucian physicians emphasized the importance of a popularization of medical knowledge and a sharing of medical resources. When asked by Huang Zhongjian why he wanted to publish a work on smallpox which he had obtained instead of keeping it a secret for his own use, Guo Yizhi replied that it should be used for the benefit of all and he dared not keep the good things from the ancients a secret.[53]

Guo was, however, not without ulterior motives for doing so. He related the story of a certain character named Xu Shumei who studied medicine, and saved the lives of many people, enabling him to obtain high achievements. Thus Guo undoubtedly also hoped that achievements in medicine would aid him in his studies and quest for office.[54] It also showed a sense of anxiety and uneasiness among the Confucian physicians concerning the many so-called secret formulas and the promulgation of the ideal of non-secrecy in the practice of medicine.

In order to counter the monopolization of special cures and secret formulas by many hereditary physicians, the Confucian physicians therefore sought to exert their own influence through the emphasis on studying (*dushu*). Thus in his preface to You Yi's *Yixue dushu ji* (Record of Studying Medicine) attacked those who did not study the classical works in medicine and thought that they could become good physicians. He praised You Yi for his diligence in studying.[55] In a similar vein, Fei Yanli in his preface to Lu Maoxiu's *Shibuzhai yishu* (Medical Works from the Shibu Studio) compared physicians to ministers, both of whom should employ *dushuren* (people who study).[56] Thus, through an emphasis on classical studies and the learned tradition, these Confucian physicians attempted to consolidate their place in the medical tradition.

Although there was no evidence of the establishment of medical schools to teach medicine in late imperial time[57], there were indications of private medical academies in some of the writings of the physicians. For example in (Medical Notes from Lüshan) by Zhang Zhicong and Gao Shichi, the preface mentioned that this was a collection of lecture notes from the *jiangtang* (lecture hall).[58]

In late imperial China, there is evidence to indicate that specialization in medicine was well-recognized with a long history of development since their separation with the *wu*. As has been shown, many Suzhou physicians, especially hereditary physicians, were specialists in one area or another. They received this knowledge mainly through the transmission of knowledge and experience from their fathers or grandfathers. The importance of specialties in medicine and the accompanying importance of experience caused much anxiety among the Confucian physicians. They could not boast of generations of practice but instead emphasized ethics and moral cultivation. This anxiety gave vitality to the discourse in medicine in late imperial China and paved the way towards a dynamic discourse on the qualifications of physicians and the efficacy of various healing traditions.

Notes

[1] The *Wenyilun*, written in 1642, has many different editions. Some of the editions, such as that of Beijing renmin chubanshe, based on the 1709 text do not have this last sentence, or mention his use of divination to decide which course to follow. Later editions revised by Liu Kui , edited by Liu Bingjin, (preface 1790 Japanese reprint 1803) have this line as well as comments by Liu Kui that this person made a living by divination, therefore he must have violated moral principles.

[2] Ibid.

[3] In the oracle bones, fish (*yu*), dates (*zao*), and mugwort (*ai*)were used as medicine to cure illnesses.

[4] Charisma here refers to the notion of authority based on a claim to a special relationship with the divine world

[5] *Lunyu, zilu* . Translation from James Legge, *The Chinese Classics* vol.1, p. 272. Another interpretation is to punctuate between *wu* and *yi*, thus becoming "If one does not have perseverance, one cannot become a shaman or a physician."

[6] Wang Fu, *Qianfulun*

[7] Zhang Congzheng was an advocate of the use of cooling therapy to treat illnesses and was known for his methods of *han* ª□ (sweating) , *xia* (purging), *tu* (emetics). There have been speculations that he only wrote the first three *juan* of the *Rumen Shiqin* but scholars have generally accepted the work to be his.

[8] For a detailed discussion on the relationship between elite and folk medicine, see Nathan Sivin, "Ailment and Cure in Traditional China: An Anthropological Study of Classical and Popular Medicine before Modern Times, with Implications for the Present."

[9] Paul Unschuld, *Medicine in China: A History of Pharmaceutics* (Berkeley: University of California Press, 1986), p. 162.

[10] Joseph Levenson, "The Amateur Ideal in Ming and Early Ch'ing Society: Evidence from Painting" in *Modern China and Its Confucian Past: The Problem of Intellectual Continuity* (New York: Anchor Books, 1964), p. 21.

[11] Ibid., p. 22.

[12] Fei Xiaotong, *China' Gentry: Essays in Rural-Urban Relations* (Chicago: University of Chicago Press, 1953), p. 74. Fei further believes that the separation of the gentry from practical technical knowledge was necessary to acquire and maintain the prestige of the gentry class. See pp. 59–74.

[13] Elman, *From Philosophy to Philology: Intellectual and Social Aspects of Change in Late Imperial China*; Dardess, *Confucianism and Autocracy: Professional Elites in the Founding of the Ming Dynasty*

[14] *Shiji, liezuan* (biographies) *juan* 45.

[15] Paul Unschuld gives a slightly different translation "For someone who believes in demons and spirits it is useless to speak of the virtues of a moral life. For someone who opposes treatment with needles and stones it is futile to speak of utmost skills." *Medicine in China: A History of Ideas*, p. 287.

[16] A work traditionally attributed to the Duke of Zhou of the Western Zhou (1122–770 B.C.) dynasty, it is a record of the institutions during the Zhou. However later scholars have disagreed on the time and authorship of the work, many attributing it to a later date.

[17] *Zhouli, Tianguan*

[18] Ibid.

[19] Sometimes also identified as *Youxiong* such as that of the physicians' guild in Suzhou. See Hong Huanchun, "Lun Ming Qing Suzhou diqu huiguan de xingzhi ji qi zuoyong" in *Zhongguoshi Yanjiu* v.2, 1980, pp. 3–15.

[20] *Huangdi neijing,*

[21] *Zhouli, Tianguan*

[22] Even though qualifying examinations for medicine began in China as discussed by Needham and Lu in "China and the Origins of Qualifying Examinations in Medicine" in *Clerks and Craftsmen in China and the West*, by Joseph Needham (Cambridge: Cambridge University Press, 1970), pp. 379–395, they were for the testing of candidates for the Imperial Academy of Medicine and never became a necessary condition for the practice of medicine in traditional China. Therefore it meant that passing the medical examinations for the Academy did not necessarily validate one's medical expertise and guarantee one a lucrative practice. If anything, students in the medical academies in the prefectural districts found themselves in a lower status than the Confucian physicians.

23 Sivin, "Ailment and Cure,"

24 Zhang Cai ,*Zhiweitang wencun* (Preserved Essays from the Zhiwei Hall), preface dated 1674, 1965 Library of Congress photocopy of the National Beijing Library edition, *wen* ñ□11:23a–25a.

25 Ibid.

26 1. *dafangmai* (general practice, adult); 2. *xiaofangmai* (pediatrics); 3. *fengke* (wind); 4. *yanke*. (eye); 5. *chuangzhong* □ (external injuries and swellings) 6. *zheshangke* (fractures); 7. *chanke*. (obstetrics); 8. *kouchi* (mouth and teeth), 9. *yanhou* (throat); 10. *zhenke* (acupuncture); 11. *jiuke* (moxa); 12. *jinzu* (incised wounds); 13. *shujinke* (divination?).

27 *Linzheng zhinan yian*, p. 649.

28 Ibid., p. 630.

29 Wang Weide , *zi* Linhong also Hongxu *hao* Linwu Shanren also Dingdingzi. He was a native of Dongting Xishan of Wu county.

30 QSG, *liejuan* 289, WXZ, *yishu liejuan*, 75a.

31 Wang Weide, *Waike Zhengzhi Quanshengji* (Preface to the Complete Works for the Diagnosis and Treatment of External Injuries) in *Zhongguo Yijikao* (A Study of Chinese Medical Texts), compiled by Tamba no Mototane, published 1826 (Beijing: Renmin weisheng chubanshe, 1983), pp. 960–961.

32 Ibid.

33 Chen was from Jiangsu Nantong ½ṇq and was famous for his work *Waike Zhengzong* (Orthodox Manual of External Illnesses), published in 1617. Chen emphasized the importance of understanding the internal causes for the external manifestations of the illnesses. He believed that all external illnesses were based upon internal causes. Although he derided some contemporary physicians who carelessly prescribed medicine and resorted to surgery rashly, he recognized the importance of surgery in medicine and in his work he listed methods for procedures such as amputations and stitching.

34 Li Jingwei and Li Zhidong , *Zhongguo gudai yixueshi lue* (An Outline of the History of Medicine in Ancient China) (Hebei: Hebei Jishu Chubanshe, 1990), p.315.

35 Ibid., pp. 314–316.

36 WXZ, 75B: 8b.

37 Ibid.

38 By *guoyi*, Zhao Xuemin was probably referring to those elite Confucian physicians.

39 *Ding,* drugs with upward action, generally referred to drugs which generally were emetics by folk physicians. *Hanying zhongyi cidian* (Chinese-English Dictionary of Traditional Chinese Medicine) edited by Ou Ming (Hong Kong: Joint Publishing [H.K.] Co., Ltd., 1988), p. 276.

40 *Chuan* , drugs with downward action, were drugs generally with purgative effects used by folk physicians. Ibid., p. 235.

41 Zhao Xuemin, *Chuanya neipian* (The Inner Essay of the Principle Book of Quackery) 1890 edition, Foreword:1.

42 Xu Dachun ,"*Zhenjiu Shichuanlun*" (Discussion on the Loss of Transmission of Acupuncture and Moxibustion) in *Yixue yuanliulun* (Topical Discussions on the History of Medicine) Preface 1757 (Beijing: Zhongguo shudian, 1987), pp. 2b–3a.

43 Ibid. Translation taken from Paul Unschuld, *Forgotten Traditions of Ancient Chinese Medicine*, p. 244.

44 Ibid., p.246.

[45] Ren Xigeng ,"Taiyiyuanzhi (An Annal of the Imperial Medical Academy," in *Qingdai zhanggu zhuilu*. (A Collection of Historical Records of the Qing Dynasty), edited by Zhou Kangxie (Chongwen shudian, 1971), p.169.

[46] For a discussion on the transmission of medical knowledge see Yamada Keiji "Igaku no denju (The transmission of medicine) in *Yorunaku tori* (Tokyo: Iwanami shoten, 1990) pp. 55–96.

[47] Dai Shigong (1324–1405) *zi* Yüanli, native of Zhejiang. He was well versed in the classics as well as astronomy and geomancy, he also was fond of studying medical works and studied under the famous physician Zhu Zhenheng. In 1386 he was called to the capital to treat the illness of Ming Taizu and was rewarded as a *yüyi* in the Imperial Medical Academy and was much respected by the emperor for his medical skills and his knowledge. He was exempt from audiences when the weather was bad. When Ming Taizu died, many imperial physicians were executed but Dai was exempted and continued to serve until 1405.

[48] Zhu Zhenheng (1281–1358) *zi*_Yanxiu , also known as Danxi ,native of present day Zhejiang province Yiwu county during the Yüan. He studied the classics and the teaching of Zhu Xi under Xu Qian and studied medicine because of his mother's illness. He later took up the study of medicine earnestly at the encouragement of Xu Qian who had contracted a serious illness. Deciding that the use of *jüfang* (written prescriptions), which was fashionable at the time and which was based to a large extent upon the work *Taiping huimin hejijüfang*, did not meet the needs of the time, he travelled widely and finally sought to study under the famous physician Luo Zhiti. Zhu then was able to read books of the northern masters of Liu Wansu, Zhang Congzheng, and Li Gao. Zhu Zhenheng was considered as the great synthesizer of medicine who related the theoretical knowledge developed in the Han to the empirical knowledge accumulated since then concerning drugs and diseases.

[49] Yang Xunji, *Sutan,* as quoted in Qian Yuanming et.al. ed. *Jinshibaijia yilu* □ (Medical Collection from the Hundred Schools in the Classics and Histories) (Hubei: Guangdong keji chubanshe, 1986), p. 286.

[50] The discussion on the four physicians began in the Ming and referred to Liu Wansu , Li Dongyuan, Zhang Conghe , and Zhu Zhenheng. There have been cases however where Zhang Ji was thought to be the Zhang in the *sidajia*. This created heated discussions where many regarded Zhang Ji as a sage and that the inclusion of him in the *sidajia* belittled the importance of his place in medical history.

[51] Ye Tianshi, *Linzhen zhinan yian* (Medical Cases for Clinical Practice) Xu Lingtai (commentary) 1959 first edition (Shanghai: Renmin chubanshe, 1976), pp. 94–95.

[52] The story also claimed that the rivalry was so deep that Xue Xue named his studio *saoye zhuang* (studio of sweeping leaves) and Ye Gui in turn used the name *taxue zhai* (stomping on snow studio). See for example biographies of Xue Xue and Ye Tianshi in MGWXZ 75b. Stories of their intense rivalry however has been called into doubt by some later physicians such as Lu Maoxiu who dismissed them as malicious rumors. Lu Maoxiu, *Shibucai yishu* (Medical Works from the Shibu Studio) 1884 edition, 11:14.

[53] Huang Zhongjian, preface of "*Xianchuan douzhen qishu* (Miraculous Book on Smallpox Passed down from the Immortals) in Guo Aichun ed. *Zhongguo fensheng yiji kao* (Study of Medical Works in China by Provinces) vol.1 (Tianjin: Kexue jishu chubanshe, 1984), pp. 772–773.

[54] Ibid.

[55] Xu Dachun, preface to *Yixue dushu ji* (Record of Studying Medicine) by You Yi. Based on 1814 edition and edited with 1884 and 1936 editions. (Beijing: Renmin weishen chubanshe, 1991), pp.1–2.

[56] Fei Yanli, preface to *Shibuzhai yishu*, pp.2–3.

[57] Shinno Reiko (2007) argues for the establishment of medical schools in association with the *sanhuang miao* in the Yuan dynasty.

[58] Zhang Zhicong and Gao Shichi, *Lüshan yichao* (Medical Notes from Lüshan), original Preface by Zhang Zhicong dated 1699 (Taibei: Tianyi chubanshe, 1973). However it is unclear whether these were the lectures of Zhang or Gao.

CONCLUSION

IN the juxtaposition of the 1229 rubbing of the *Pingjiang Tubei* (stone rubbing of Pingjiang), and the 1945 aerial photograph of Suzhou, Frederick Mote presented the stability in physical form of the city.[1] However this masked the vibrant changes that had taken place within the region in terms of culture and economics, and medicine was one of the important fields that witnessed tremendous developments. This book is a study of the dynamics of change and transformation in the medical landscape in late imperial China in the Jiangnan region. The vibrant economic and cultural developments in Jiangnan led to a dynamic discourse on legitimation among the different groups of physicians that became especially significant as more scholars joined the ranks. Since the late imperial Chinese state did not set up licensing laws, and there was little regulation over the practice of medicine by the state, these debates served as ways of negotiating boundaries and establishing legitimation for the practice of medicine. The lack of licensing laws, however, did not mean that the state was uninterested in medicine. On the contrary, the legitimacy of the state and the ruler was tied to their ability to provide care for the people and show benevolence in times of need. Patronage of medicine was, therefore, part of the state's strategy in enhancing her authority. This was accomplished through sponsoring publications, setting up charitable pharmacies, and patronizing the recognized orthodox tradition of the Three Emperors through temple worship. Medicine is nevertheless a technical skill responding to very real practical needs. This reality led to the emergence of competing schools that have evolved different methods of therapy based on differing views of disease, environment, and the body. This difference became especially sharp in late imperial times when several large-scale epidemics ravaged regions of China.

Physicians in late imperial China, though officially labeled as artisans and placed under such a category in the local gazetteers and historical biographies, nevertheless possessed a certain "professional charisma" which the other artisans did not share. This "professional charisma" was closely related to their perceived power of healing, and thus an assumed power over death.[2] The legitimacy of their power over the biological body was based upon both the moral and symbolic power ascribed to them by the Confucian doctrines, and upon the accumulation of practical knowledge through experience which they possessed.

Suzhou physicians in late imperial China were not a homogeneous group. Unlike physicians today who can clearly be distinguished as a politically and socially dominant professional group with clear guidelines for admission, and regulations concerning acceptable conduct for its members, the physicians in Suzhou did not form a professional group in this sense, nor did they exert much social and political power. However I have argued that the idea of professionalization is useful in looking at these late imperial physicians because there was a growing sense of identity among them, fostered by the imbricated relationship with the intellectual community and the publishing networks. The influx of elites into the ranks of physicians in late imperial China also brought about an effort to renegotiate the boundaries of legitimacy, and attempts were made to demarcate more clearly the lines of inclusion into the group.

Traditional Chinese medicine was and is a dynamic discipline constantly undergoing a process of redefinition and change. The emerging dominance of the *wenbing* (warm factor) school in late imperial Jiangnan was representative of such a trend. It was not only an effort in the search for a better treatment of epidemic diseases which ravaged large portions of the population, but it was also stimulated by the interests in the re-examination of classical medical texts. This latter trend was very much related to the evidential research movement which influenced many in the intellectual community. The careful study of the classical works such as Zhang Ji's *Shanghanlun* (Treatise on Cold Damaged Disorders) brought about new ideas on the diagnosis and treatment of diseases.

While in my book I have concentrated on mainly the elite physicians and their attempts to formulate an identity within the society, we should not forget that they do not represent the whole of the medical tradition. From the discussions among the physicians and cases of patients, it is quite clear that very often the elite and folk traditions were both employed in an effort to cure an illness. Prayers to spirits and gods, charms, and amulets were not uncommon and even some of the elite physicians advocated some of these measures when they seemed to be unable to effect a cure. Thus even the Emperor Kangxi ordered prayers to be said for his mother when she was ill and ordered any priests or monks known to be skilled in curing illnesses to be sent immediately.[3]

The actual efficacy of the treatments is difficult to gauge, and the impact that medicine had on the health of the population is subject to debate. Though there was widespread dissemination of medical knowledge through the printing of medical books, it was probably in the care of children that medical knowledge made a difference. Susan Mann speculates that "The most important effect of increased access to medical texts in the early Ch'ing period was arguably the dissemination of knowledge about the healthful benefits of proper breast feeding for children."[4]

It was probably the general lack of confidence in physicians that the phenomenon of consultation of several physicians at one time occurred. As we have seen, this led to bitter complaints by the physicians. This situation, however, was not very different from that in Europe during the seventeenth, eighteenth, and nineteenth centuries when the sick typically tried to "sample more and more sorts of doctors and medicine, even indulging in a 'try anything' approach, which might be dignified with the appellation of the 'experimental method', or more honestly, be viewed as the triumph of hope over experience."[5] The wealthy Suzhou patient could certainly identify with the way in which the wealthy in Europe approached medicine: "Those who could afford to do so, frequently drew upon a wide range of *regular* physicians, seeking second, third, and fourth opinions, and showing no compunction about also sampling the therapies and the drugs of empirics."[6] The patients themselves, and the patients' families, were often knowledgeable about methods of diagnosis and medicine. Therefore interference was not uncommon and was another major concern of the physicians.

Undoubtedly some of the medicine helped alleviate the pains and sufferings and there were highly skilled surgeons. Yet when there was the consultation of many physicians, and the change of prescriptions changed when there was no immediate improvement in the patient's condition, then it was doubtful whether any of the prescriptions would have been of much use. Medical knowledge was considered an essential knowledge and self-diagnosis was not uncommon. If the physicians complained about their patients, the patients were also dissatisfied with the physicians. The Kangxi emperor himself was very interested in medicine and often dispatched Imperial Academy physicians and special medicine for his high officials. However Kangxi was highly critical of the physicians: "The trouble with so many of today's doctors is that they claim to have various marvelous prescriptions that have been handed down in the family, that'll cure all sorts of sickness, and they dispense them at random. Yet you can see that even they have their doubts as to their efficacy, since they will give one prescription and then follow it with a whole lot of others—but if the first was any good why do they need these extra ones? Few of them have the intelligence or the critical skills shown in the Yellow Emperor's *Classic of Internal Medicine*. Also their teaching is shallow, and I've read enough in the medical literature to know when their claims to true antiquity are spurious. They don't keep up their studies of the pulses, they ignore relevant case histories, they distinguish between their rich and poor patients, and they concentrate on the hunt for fame and money. Often they don't know the basic principles of medicine, they tend to ask wild questions and make wild statements, sometimes even inventing prescriptions that really harm people. I know this well, and it makes me sad, but I can't prevent it. One can't prosecute all the doctors who have a little business and wander from place to place, just managing to stay alive."[7]

The physicians in late imperial Jiangnan operated within a highly commercialized and monetarized society. This also meant that they had to be innovative in a consumer society. In order to gain patients, especially wealthy patients, mere proclamation of a moral superiority and the possession of benevolence would not be useful for a physician to gain many patients. What was important was for him to advertise himself and build up a reputation. This could be accomplished by the recommendation of successful cases and by the compilation of *yian* (medical cases) in which most of the cases recorded were ones which the physician had successfully cured. Medicine, when pursued properly, was a lucrative enterprise.

The flourishing of trade both internal and foreign meant that mobility was relatively easy. There was a lucrative trade with Japan which also included many medical works and had a significant impact on the development of medicine in the country. Physicians from Suzhou were also found to have travelled to Japan. One Wu Dainan unfortunately died shortly after he arrived. Other physicians who were active were Zhu Laizhang and Zhou Qilai . Zhu had traveled to Japan several times.[8] In 1725 both of his elder brothers Zhu Peizhang and Zhu Zizhang accompanied him. The Qing Yongzheng emperor (1723–35) at the time was concerned with piracy and efforts to circumvent regulations along the coast, especially with Japan. Therefore Zhu Laizhang found himself recruited as an informer.[9] Zhu was not, however, recorded in any of the biographical sources and evidently not considered worthy of inclusion into the ranks of physicians.

The introduction of Western medicine into China began with the Jesuits during the sixteenth-century. At the beginning their influence was limited to areas such as Macao where they set up hospitals to treat patients. The earliest Suzhou physician to take note of Western medicine was Wang Honghan, a physician who had converted to Catholicism. Western medicine at the time did not make much of an impact on traditional medicine. It was not until during the mid-nineteenth century that saw the influx of missionaries into China and hospitals were set up within China. The first Western style hospital was set up in Suzhou in 1877.[10] Most of the later hospitals were established by Western missionaries. The last years of the Qing government saw efforts to learn Western techniques, including medicine. A group of students were sent abroad to study medicine and included several students from Suzhou.[11]

Western medicine came to be seen as a necessary aspect of modernization and traditional medicine, together with Confucianism, came to be seen as baggage that hindered the process of the creation of a new country capable of resisting Western imperialism. It would be another project to explore the relationship between the introduction of Western concepts of illness and health, and "scientific medicine" with the attempt in China to strengthen itself, and to explore the correspondence between the curing of the biological body and the social body.

However in the effort to "scientize" and "rationalize" traditional Chinese medicine, some Chinese scholars have been eager to purge classical texts of all sections deemed "superstitious." The teaching of Chinese medicine is also combined with techniques of Western biomedicine. Acupuncture has come to represent Traditional Chinese Medicine (TCM) in the West, and the representation of the body has been based on the anatomical model rather than the cosmological body in classical medicine.

Notes

[1] Frederick Mote, "A Millennium of Chinese Urban History: Form, Time, and Space Concepts in Soochow," in *Rice University Studies*, 59.4 (1973):35–65.

[2] For a discussion on the "professional charisma" of doctors, see J. Kosa, "Entrepreneurship and Charisma in the Medical Profession," in *Social Science and Medicine*, 4 (1970): 25–40.

[3] *Suzhou Zhizao Li Xu Zouzhe* (Memorials of the Suzhou Superintendent of Imperial Silk Manufacturing Li Xu), p. 236.

[4] Susan Mann, "Women, Families, and Gender Relations," in *The Cambridge History of China*, v.9, ed. by Willard J. Peterson, p. 445.

[5] Roy Porter, *Health for Sale: Quackery in England 1660–1850* (Manchester: Manchester University Press, 1989), p.24.

[6] Ibid.

[7] Quotation taken from Jonathan D. Spence, *Emperor of China, Self Portrait of K'ang-hsi* (New York: Vintage Books, 1988), pp.99–100.

[8] Oba Osamu (Record of Chinese Ships Coming into Harbor) Kansai Daigaku Tozai Gakujutsu Kenkyûjo, 1974, pp. 44–55.

[9] *Yongzheng Zhupi Yuzhi* (Vermillion Edicts of the Yongzheng Emperor), v. 42, p.14b–15a.

[10] Yu Lian, "Bainianlai Suzhou Xiyi Shiye Gaikuang" (A Brief Account of Western Medicine in Suzhou in Recent Hundred Years) in *Suzhou Shizhi* (Record of the History of Suzhou), vol.2, 1990, p. 103.

[11] Ibid., p. 106.

GLOSSARY

Aitang Yihua 藹堂醫話
anmo boshi 按摩博士
bagua 八卦
Bai shi *xuepai* 白氏學派
Ban Gu 班固
Baopuzi 抱朴子
beitianfang 悲田坊
bencao 本草
Bencao Gangmu 本草綱目
Bian Que 扁鵲
Bian Que xuepai 扁鵲學派
bianming shanghan shiyi 辨明傷寒時疫
Bogao 伯高
Boxiang 柏鄉
boxue hongci 博學鴻詞
bu 卜
bubidu 不必讀
Bushi Zhengzhong 卜筮正宗
buwei liangxiang, ji wei liangyi 不為良相, 即為良醫
Chang Sang Jun 長桑君
Changmen 閶門
Changshu 常熟
Changzhou 長州
chanke 產科
Changsha 長沙
Chao Yüanfang 巢元方
Chen Chuanzhuo 陳傳倬
Chen Nianzu 陳念祖(Xiuyuan 修園)
Chen Shigong 陳實功
Chenghuang ci 城隍祠
Chenghuang miao 城隍廟
cirepian 刺熱篇
Chongren *xian* 崇仁縣
chuan 串
chuangzhong 瘡腫
Chuanya neipian 串雅內篇
Chunyu Yi 淳于意
Cuncunzhai yihua gao 存存齋醫話稿
dafangmai 大方脈
Dai Yuanli 戴元禮
dayi 大疫
daxue 大學
Deng Mingyuan 鄧明遠
deyi 德醫
dianke 典科
dianyuguan 典獄官
ding 頂
diwang miao 帝王廟
dongwen 冬溫
du 黷
dushu 讀書
erke 兒科
Fan Zhongyan 范仲淹
Fang Yizhi 方以智
fangji 方技
fanglun 方論
fangshi 方士

fangshiyi 方士醫
fangxu 防虛
fanli 凡例
Fei Yanli 費延釐
Feng Guifen 馮桂芬
fengke 風科
Feng Xie 馮燮
Fenghou 風后
fengwen 風溫
Fu Weikang 傅維康
Fu Yunke 傅允科
fu 府
fu 腑
Fugongsheng 副貢生
fugu pai 復古派
fuke 婦科
fuqi wenbing 伏氣溫病
Fuxi 伏犧
fuzi miao 夫子廟
Gao Shizong 高士宗
Gao Wu 高武
Gao Zhongxian 高忠憲
Gao Ziyuan 高紫垣
Ge Hong 葛洪 (*Baopuzi* 抱朴子)
gedawen 疙瘩瘟
gexin pai 革新派
gong 工
gongsuo 公所
Goumang 勾芒
Gu Jiegang 顧頡剛
Gu Jingyuan 顧靖遠 (Songyuan 松園)
Guangfu *zhen* 光福鎮
guansong boshi 關送博士
Guiyuqu 鬼于區
Gujin yitong daquan 古今醫統大全
guoyi 國醫
Guo Yizhi 過繹之
Gusu 姑蘇
guwen 古文
Hanshu 漢書
he 和
Hejian xuepai 河間學派
houke 喉科
houtian 後天
Hua Tuo 華佗
Huainanzi 淮南子
Huang Liuhong 黃六鴻
Huang Yuanyu 黃元御
Huang Zhongjian 黃中堅
Huangdi 黃帝
Huangdi bashiyi nanjing 黃帝八十一難經
Huangdi neijing 黃帝內經
Huangdi neijing suwen 黃帝內經素問
Huangdi xuepai 黃帝學派
Huangdi zhenjiu 黃帝針灸
Huangfu Mi 皇甫謐
Huating 華亭
huiantang 惠安堂
huiguan 會館
huimin yaoju 惠民薬局
Jiading 嘉定
Ji'an lu sanhuang miao tian ji 吉安路三皇廟田記
Jiang Pu 蔣溥
Jiangnan 江南
jiangtang 講堂
Jiangxi 江西
Jiankang lu sanhuang miao ji 健康路三皇廟記
Jiao Xun 焦循
jiedu 解毒
Jinhua 金華
Jin Yuan sidajia 金元四大家
Jin Zhao 斤照
Jingde chongsheng neidian 景德重聖內殿
Jinghui dian 景惠殿
Jingluo gejue 經絡歌訣
Jingluo xuedao ge 經絡穴道歌
jinkui 金匱
Jinkui yaolue 金匱要略
jinshi 進士
jinwen 今文
Jinze 金澤
jinzu 金鏃
jitian liji yi kai wanshi jiaohua zi yuan 繼天立極以開萬世教化之源
jiu chuan 九傳
jiu zhe bi er cheng yi 九折臂而成醫

Jiudaiji 就貸季
jiuke 灸科
jiupin 九品
jiyi 疾醫
ju fang 局方
jun you ji yin yao chen xian chang zhi, qing you ji yin yao zi xian chang zhi 君有疾飲葯臣先嘗之、親有疾飲葯子先嘗之
juren 舉人
juye 舉業
Kang Zuolin 康作霖
Kangxi 康熙
kaozheng 考證
Ke Qin 柯琴 (Yunbo 韻伯)
Kong Yingda 孔穎達
Kongzi miao 孔子廟
kouchi 口齒
Kunshan 昆山
laofang 老方
laoyi shaobu 老醫少卜
Lei Dasheng 雷大升 (Yunshang 允上)
Leigong 雷公
Lenglu yihua bupian 冷盧醫話補篇
Li Gao 李杲 (Mingzhi 明之, *hao* Dongyuan 東垣)
Li Shizhen 李時珍
Li Xu 李煦
Li Yuchun 李雨春
Li Zhongzi 李中梓 (Shicai 士材)
li 禮
liang 兩
libu shilang 禮部侍郎
libu 禮部
Liji zhengyi 禮記正義
Liji 禮記
Lindeng 林嶝
Lin Tao 臨洮
Lin Yi 林億
Lingshu 靈樞
lingyi 鈴醫
liqi 癘氣
Liu Wansu 劉完素 (Shouzhen 守真)
liujing 六經
liuyi 流醫
liuyin 六淫
Loujiang 婁江
lu 路
Lu Maoxiu 陸懋修 (Jiuzhi 九芝)
Lu Song 陸嵩
Lu Yitian 陸以湉
Lu Zhenming 吕震名
Lunyu 論語
Lüshan yichao 侶山醫鈔
Lüshi chunqiu 呂氏春秋
Ma Shihuang 馬師皇
Ma Shu 馬俶(Yuanyi 元儀)
Mahuang 麻黃
Mei Wending 梅文鼎
menhu 門戶
Mawangdui 馬王堆
Mengzi 孟子
Miao Zunyi 繆遵義 (Fangyan 方彥)
mifang 秘方
Ming-Qing jinshit timingzhuan 明清進士提名傳
Minguo Wuxian zhi 民國吳縣志
mingyi 明醫
Mingyi zazhu 明醫雜著
mingyi 名醫
Miyazaki Ichisada 宮崎市定
Mohai jinhu 墨海金壺
nanbeihuo ye 南北貨業
nangyong 囊廱
Nanjing 難經
nanpujitang 男普濟堂
neike 内科
Nenggai zhai manlu 能改齋漫錄
Ni Changyu 倪長玗
Niu Ruolin 牛若麟
nüyi 女醫
Peng Shaosheng 彭紹升
ping 平
ping rebinglun 評熱病論
Pingjiang *fu* 平江府
Pingjiang *lu* 平江路
Pingjiang tubei 平江圖碑
pujitang 普濟堂
Qianfu lun 潛夫論
Qiantang 錢塘

Qiao Xinyu 喬心宇
Qiao Zongfu 喬宗甫
Qibo 岐伯
Qin Yueren 秦越人
qingre 清熱
Quli 曲禮
relun 熱論
renshu 仁術
renzheng 仁政
Rumen shiqin 儒門事親
ruyi 儒醫
san 散
sanbao 三寶
san zhe gong zhi wei liang yi 三折肱知為良醫
sanfen 三墳
sanhuang miao 三皇廟
sanhuang wudi 三皇五帝
sanshi 三世
Shanghai 上海
shanghan 傷寒
Shanghan laisuji 傷寒來蘇集
Shanghanlun 傷寒論
shangshi 上士
Shao Yu 少俞
Shao Yong 邵雍
shaolao 少牢
Shaoshi 少師
sheju shiyao 設局施薬
Shexian 歙縣
Shen Douyuan 申斗垣
Shen Kuo 沈括
Shen Laiheng 沈來亨
Shen Shiyu 沈時譽
shen wu qi ye 慎物齊也
sheng 聖
Shengji *dian* 聖濟殿
Shennong bencao 神農本草
Shennong bencao jing 神農本草經
Shennong 神農
shi 史
Shisan jing zhushu 十三經註疏
shiyi 世醫
shiyi 時醫
shiyi 食醫
Shi Yousheng 施幼聲
Shibuzhai yishu 世補齋醫書
Shiji 史記
shiwen 濕溫
shizhe 十哲
shouhui 收回
shouyi 獸醫
shujinke 書禁科
Shun 舜
sidajia 四大家
Siku quanshu zongmu tiyao 四庫全書總目提要
Sima Qian 司馬遷
Siqi tiaoshen dalunpian 四氣調神大論篇
sisheng 四聖
Song Yingxing 宋應星
Songben 宋本
Songjiang 松江
Su Shi 蘇軾
Su Tiege 蘇鐵戈
Sun Qi 孫奇
Sun Simiao 孫思邈
Sunu maijue 素女脈訣
Sutan 蘇談
Suwen maijue 素問脈訣
Suwen 素問
Suzhou 蘇州
Taichang si 太常寺
Taiping shenghui fang 太平聖惠方
taiyiyuan 太醫院
Tamba no Mototane 丹波元胤
Tang Dalie 唐大烈(Lisan 立三, *hao* Lisan 笠三)
Tang hui yao 唐會要
tang shang guan 堂上官
tang 堂
Tang Xueji 唐學吉
tangyao 湯藥
Tao Hongjing 陶弘景
taxue zhai 踏雪齋
Tianbao 天寶
Tianguan Zhongzai 天官冢宰
tiju 提舉
Tongjun 桐君
tongxue 同學

tu 徒
Tu Xuan 屠璇
tuiguan 推官
tuina 推拿
waigan wenrebing 外感溫熱病
waike 外科
Waike Qixuan 外科啓玄
Waike zhengzhi quanshengji 外科証治全生集
Waike zhunsheng 外科準繩
wan 丸
Wang Ang 汪昂
Wang Bing 王冰 (Qixuanzi 啓玄子)
Wang Fu 王符
Wang Guangjue 汪光爵
Wang Honghan 王宏翰 (Huiyuan 惠源, Haoranzi 浩然子)
Wang Kentang 王肯堂 (Yutai 宇泰)
Wang Lun 王綸
Wang Ruogu 王若谷
Wang Shixiong 王士雄 (Mengying 孟英)
Wang Shuhe 王叔和
Wang Wei 王禕
Wang Weide 王維德 (Linhong 林洪)
Wang Xilie 王希烈
Wang Yuanshi 汪元軾
Wang Zijie 王子接 (Pusan 普三)
Wang Zhongguang 王仲光
Wei Cicang 韋慈藏
Wei Litong 魏荔彤
wei 衛, *qi* 氣, *ying* 營, *xue* 血
Wei Shanjun 韋善俊
Weiyutang 位育堂
wenbing 溫病
wendu 溫毒
Weng Jieshou 翁介壽
Wenhua dian 文華殿
wennue 溫瘧
Wenyilun 瘟疫論
wenxuan 文宣
Wu 吳
Wu Cheng 吳澄
Wu Dainan 吳戴南
Wu Qian 吳謙
Wu Tang 吳塘 (Jutong 鞠通)
Wu Youxing 吳有性 (Youke 又可)
wu 巫
Wucheng 烏程
Wujiang 吳江
Wujing zhengyi 五經正義
Wuxian 吳縣
wuyi 巫醫
Wuyi huijiang 吳醫匯講
wuyun liuqi 五運六氣
Wuzhong yian 吳中醫案
Wuzhong 吳中
xian 縣
xiangyan puji 香喦普濟
xiantian 先天
Xiao Jing 蕭京
xiao 孝
xiaodao 小道
xiaofangmai 小方脈
xiashi 下士
Xilei tang 錫類堂
xingming zai yu yishu zhe 姓名載於醫書者
Xu Chunfu 徐春甫
Xu Dachun 徐大椿 (Lingtai 靈胎, also Huixi laoren 洄溪老人)
Xu Guoqi 許國器
Xu Xiaobiao 徐孝標
xuanyong 懸廱
Xue Xue 薛雪 (Shengbai 生白)
xue 學
xunke 訓科
xuntao 熏陶
yanke 眼科
Yan Song 嚴嵩
Yang Jizhou 楊繼洲
Yang Xunji 楊循吉
yangbing fang 養病坊
yangji yuan 養濟院
yangke 瘍科
yangmaowen 羊毛瘟
yangsheng 養生
yangshi 陽實
yangyi 瘍醫
Yangzhou 揚州
yanhou 咽喉

yanke 眼科
Yao 堯
yaosi 藥肆
yaowang miao 藥王廟
Ye Gui 葉桂 (Tianshi 天士, Xiangyan 香岩, Nanyang xiansheng 南陽先生)
Yi Yin 伊尹
yi 義
yi xiao wei gui, yi tuo wei wei 以消為貴、以托為畏
yian 醫案
yibusanshi bufuqiyao 醫不三世 不服其藥
yihua 醫話
Yihuang xian sanhuang miao ji 宜黃縣三皇廟記
yili 疫厲
yijing 醫經
Yin Shidan 殷士儋
yinci 淫祠
yinxu 陰虛
yinyi 淫醫
yinyi 隱醫
yinzheng 陰症
yirentang 一仁堂
yisheng 醫生
yisheng 醫聖
yishi 醫史
yishi 醫師
yishu 藝術
Yishui xuepai 易水學派
yiwang miao 醫王廟
yiwen 藝文
yixue boshi 醫學博士
Yixue congshu 醫學叢書
Yixue congzhong lu 醫學從衆錄
Yixue dushu ji 醫學讀書記
yixue zhengke 醫學正科
yizhai 醫齋
yizhe zuojiao, qiongjia budao 醫者坐轎，窮家不到
yizheng 疫症
Yizong bidu 醫宗必讀
Yizong jinjian 醫宗金鑑
yongyi 庸醫
Yongyuan ju 永元局
You Cheng 尤乘 (Shengzhou 生洲)
You Yi 尤怡 (Zaijing 在涇, Sihe Shanren 飼鶴山人)
youxiong 有熊
Yu Chang 喻昌(Jiayan 嘉言)
Yu Fu 俞跗
Yu Ji 虞集
Yu Mingjian 俞明鑑
Yu Shiyue 俞士悅
Yu Zonghai 俞宗海
Yüan Chengzong 元成宗
Yuanhe 元和
Yuanmiao guan 圓妙觀
Yunjian 雲間
yunqi 運氣
yuying tang 育嬰堂
zalu 雜錄
zang 臟
Zhang Chai 張釵
Zhang Congzheng 張從正 (Zihe 子和)
Zhang Deng 張登
Zhang Ji 張機 (Zhongjing 仲景)
Zhang Jiebin 張介賓 (Jingyue 景岳)
Zhang Jingtao 張景燾
Zhang Lu 張璐 (Luyü 路玉, Shiwan Laoren 石頑老人)
Zhang Xuecheng 章學誠
Zhang Yüansu 張元素 (Jiegu 潔古)
Zhang Zai 張載
Zhang Zhuo 張倬
zhangli 瘴癘
Zhangshi yitong 張氏醫通
Zhao Qingchu 趙晴初
Zhao Rujin 趙儒縉
Zhao Xuemin 趙學敏
Zhao You 趙酉
Zhejiang 浙江
zhenfa 診法
zhenjiu tongren 針灸銅人
zhenke 針科
Zheng Jian 鄭堅
Zheng Jinsheng 鄭金生
Zheng Renyuan 鄭任原
Zheng Xuan 鄭玄
zhengke 正科

Zhenjiang 鎮江
zhenjiu 針灸
Zhenjiu dacheng 針灸大成
Zhenjiu juying 針灸聚英
zheshangke 折傷科
Zhengtong zhenjiu tongren 正統針灸銅人
zhiye 職業
zhongfeng 中風
Zhongguo yixueshi 中國醫學史
zhongshuju 種樹局
Zhongyong 中庸
Zhou Qilai 周岐來
Zhou Yangjun 周揚俊 (Yüzai 禹載)
zhou 州
zhoufang 走方
zhoujin boshi 咒禁博士
Zhouli 周禮
Zhu Gong 朱肱
Zhu Laizhang 朱來章
Zhu Peizhang 朱佩章
zhusheng 諸生
Zhu Xi 朱熹
Zhu Zizhang 朱子章
zhuyou 祝由
Zhu Zhenheng 朱震亨 (Yanxiu 彥修, Danxi 丹溪)
Zhurong 祝融
Zou Bin 鄒彬
zuotang 坐堂

BIBLIOGRAPHY

Agren, Hans. "Empiricism and Speculation in Traditional East Asian Medicine," *Nihon ishigaku zasshi* 日本醫學史雜誌 (Journal of the Japan Society of Medical History) 23:2 (April 1977): 300–317.

Alford, William P. *To Steal a Book is an Elegant Offense: Intellectual Property Law in Chinese Civilization*. Stanford: Stanford University Press, 1995.

Andrews, Bridie. "Traditional Chinese Medicine as Invented Tradition." *Bulletin of the British Association for Chinese Studies* 6 (1995)

Atwell, William S. "Another Look at Silver Imports into China, ca 1635–1644." *Journal of World History* 16.4 (2005): 467–489

Beattie, Hilary. *Land and Lineage in China: A Study of T'ung-Ch'eng County in the Ming and Ch'ing Dynasties*. Cambridge: Cambridge University Press,1979.

Biagioli, Mario. *Galileo, Courtier: The Practice of Science in the Culture of Absolutism.* Chicago: University of Chicago Press, 1993.

Bodde, Derk and Clarence Morris. *Law in Imperial China: Exemplified by 190 Ch'ing Dynasty Cases*. Philadelphia: University of Pennsylvania Press,1967.

Bol, Peter K. *"This Culture of Ours" : Intellectual Transitions in T'ang and Sung China*. Stanford: Stanford University Press, 1992.

Browkaw, Cynthia. *The Ledgers of Merit and Demerit: Social Change and Moral Order in Late Imperial China*. Princeton: Princeton University Press,1991.

Buell, Paul D. "The Yin-Shan Cheng-Yao, A Sino-Uighur Dietary: Synopsis, Problems, Prospects," *Approaches to Traditional Chinese Medical Literature: Proceedings of An International Symposium on Translation Methodologies and Terminologies,* ed. by Paul Unschuld. Boston: Kluwer Academic Publishers, 1989: pp.109–127.

Cao, Bingzhang 曹炳章. *Zhongguo yixue dacheng* 中國醫學大成 (A Comprehensive Collection of Chinese Medical Works). 6v. Changsha: Yuelu shushe chubanshe, 1990.

——— *Zhongguo yixue dacheng xupian* 中國醫學大成續篇 (Supplementary of the Comprehensive Collection of Chinese Medical Works). 10 v. Changsha: Yuelu shushe chubanshe, 1992.

Cass, Victoria B. "Female Healers in the Ming and the Lodge of Ritual and Ceremony." *Journal of the American Oriental Society*. 101 (1986): 233–240.

Chang, Chung-li. *The Chinese Gentry: Studies on Their Role in Nineteenth-Century Chinese Society*. 3rd printing. Seattle: University of Washington Press, 1967.

——— *The Income of the Chinese Gentry*. Seattle: University of Washington Press, 1962.

Changzhou xianzhi. 長州縣志 (Gazetteer of Changzhou county). 1753 edition. Nanjing: Jiangsu guji chubanshe,1991.

Chen, Bangxian 陳邦賢. *Zhongguo yixueshi* 中國醫學史 (A History of Chinese Medicine) Taibei: Yuandong tushu gongshi, 1956.

Chen, Daojin 陳道瑾 and Xue Weitao 薛渭濤. *Jiangsu lidai yirenzhi* 江蘇歷代醫人志 (Collection of Jiangsu Physicians from Successive Dynasties). Nanjing: Jiangsu kexue jishu chubanshe, 1985.

Chen, Lifu 陳立夫. *Zhonghua yiyao xueshi* 中華醫藥學史(The History of Medicine in China). Taibei: The Commercial Press, 1982.

Chen, Xiuyuan 陳修園. *Yixue congzonglu* 醫學從眾錄(Record of Medicine for the Masses). Fuzhou: Fujian kexue jishu chubanshe, 1987.

——— *Yixue sanzijing* 醫學三字經 (Three-word Primer for Medicine). Author preface 1804. 12th printing. Shanghai: Shanghai kexue jishu chubanshe, 1991.

Chongzhen Wuxian zhi 崇禎吳縣志 (Gazetter of Wu County compiled in the Chongzhen reign 1628–1644). 5v. Shanghai: Shanghai shudian, 1990.

Chow, Kai-wing. "Purist Hermeneutics and Ritualist Ethics in Mid-Ch'ing Thought," *Cosmology, Ontology, and Human Efficacy: Essays in Chinese Thought*, ed. by Richard J. Smith and D.W.K. Kwok. Honolulu: University of Hawaii Press, 1993: 179–204.

Chu Ping-yi, "Song, Ming zhi ji de yishi yu ruyi" 宋、明之際的醫史與"儒醫" (Narrations of Histories of Medicine from the Song to the Ming and the Rise of the Confucian Physician) in *The Bulletin of the Institute of History and Philology, Academia Sinica*, vol. 77, Part 3 (2006)：401–449.

Croizier, Ralph. *Traditional Medicine in Modern China: Science, Nationalism, and the Tensions of Cultural Change*. Cambridge: Harvard University Press, 1968.

Cullen, Christopher. "New Windows on Chinese Medicine: Sickness and Healing in a Sixteenth-century Novel." The Joseph Needham Lecture. May 2, 1991.

Da Ming hui dian 大明會典 (DMHD) (Collected Statues and Precedents in the Great Ming). Wanli edition. Taibei: Dongnan shubaoshe, 1964.

Da Qing hui dian 大清會典 (DQHD) (Collected Statues and Precedents in the Great Qing). Qianlong preface. Taibei: Dongnan shubaoshe.

Dardess, John W. *Confucianism and Autocracy: Professional Elites in the Founding of the Ming Dynasty*. Berkeley: University of California Press,1983.

Dennerline, Jerry. *The Chia-Ting Loyalists: Confucian Leadership and Social Change in Seventeenth-Century China*. New Haven: Yale University Press,1981.

Dingwall, Robert and Philip Lewis ed. *The Sociology of The Professions: Lawyers, Doctors and Others*. London: MacMillan Press Ltd., 1983.

Du, Congming 杜聰明. *Zhongxi yixue shilue* 中西醫學史略 (An Outline of the History of Chinese and Western Medicine) Taibei: Zhonghua dadian bianinhui,1966.

Duan, Benluo 段本洛 and Zhang Qifu 張圻福. *Suzhou shougongye shi* 蘇州手工業史 (History of Handicraft Industries in Suzhou). Nanjing: Jiangsu guji chubanshe, 1986.

Dunstan, Helen. "The Late Ming Epidemics: A Preliminary Survey." *Ch'ing-shih wen-t'i* 3.3(1975): 1–59.

Duara, Prasenjit. *Culture, Power, and The State: Rural North China, 1900–1942*. Stanford: Stanford University Press, 1988.

——— "Superscribing Symbols: The Myth of Guandi, Chinese God of War." *Journal of Asian Studies* 47.4 (Nov. 1988): 778–95.

Elman, Benjamin A. *From Philosophy to Philology: Intellectual and Social Aspects of Change in Late Imperial China*. Cambridge: Harvard University Press, 1984.

——— *Classicism, Politics, and Kinship: The Ch'ang-Chou School of New Text Confucianism in Late Imperial China*. Berkeley: University of California Press, 1990.

——— *On Their Own Terms: Science in China, 1550–1900*. Cambridge: Harvard University Press, 2005.

——— and Alexander Woodside ed. *Education and Society in Late Imperial China, 1600–1900*. Berkeley: University of California Press, 1994.

Elvin, Mark. *The Pattern of the Chinese Past*. Stanford: Stanford University Press, 1973.

Ershiliushi yijia zhuanji xinzhu 二十六史醫家傳記新註(New Annotation of the Biographies of Physicians in the Twenty-six Histories). Shenyang: Liaoning University Press, 1986.

Esherick, Joseph W. and Mary B. Rankin ed. *Chinese Local Elites and Patterns of Dominance*. Berkeley: University of California Press, 1990.

Fan, Jinmin 范金民. "Qing qianqi Suzhou nongye jingji di tese" 清前期蘇州農業經濟的特色 (The Characteristics of Agricultural Economy in Suzhou during the Early Qing). *Zhongguo nongshi* 中國農史(*Chinese Agriculture*) 12:1 (1993): 46–51.

Fan, Xingzhun 范行準. *Zhongguo yixue shilue* 中國醫學史略 (An Outline of the History of Medicine in China). Beijing: Zhongyi guji chubanshe, 1986.

——— Zhongguo yufang yixue sixiangshi 中國預防醫學思想史 (A History of Preventive Medicine in China). Beijing: Renmin chubanshe,1955.

Farquhar, Judith. "Problems of Knowledge in Contemporary Chinese Medical Discourse," *Social Science and Medicine*, 24.12 (1987): 1013–1021.

Fei, Xiaotong. *China's Gentry: Essays in Rural-Urban Relations*. Chicago: University of Chicago Press,1953.

Foucault, Michel. *The Birth of the Clinic: An Archaeology of Perception*, translated by A.M.Sheridan Smith. New York: Vintage Books, 1973.

——— *Power/Knowledge: Selected Interviews and other writings 1972–1977*, ed. by Colin Gordon, translated by Colin Gordon, Leo Marshall, John Mepham and Kate Soper. New York: Pantheon Books,1977.

Freidson, Eliot. *Profession of Medicine: A Study of the Sociology of Applied Knowledge*. New York: Dodd, Mead & Company, 1970.

Fu, Weikang 傅維康. *Zhongguo yixueshi* 中國醫學史 (A History of Medicine in China). Shanghai: Xinhua shudian, 1990.

Fuma, Susumu 夫馬進. "Minshin jidai no soshi to soshô seido" 明清時代の訟師と訴訟制度 (Pettifoggers and the Litigation System in Ming and Qing). *Chûgoku kinsei no hôsei to shakai* 中國近世の法制と社會(Society and the Legal System in Modern China).Kyoto: Institute for Research in Humanities at Kyoto University, 1993: pp.437–483.

Furth, Charlotte. "Concepts of Pregnancy, Childbirth ,and Infancy in Ch'ing Dynasty China." *Journal of Asian Studies*, 46.1 (February 1987): 7–35.

——— *A Flourishing Yin: Gender in China's Medical History, 960–1665*. Berkeley: University of California Press, 1999.

Ge Hong 葛洪. *Alchemy, Medicine, Religion in the China of A.D. 320: The Nei P'ien of Ko Hung (Pao-p'utzu)*. Translated by James R. Ware. Massachusetts: The M.I.T. Press, 1966; Taiwan reprinted edition, Taipei: Southern Materials Center, 1984.

Goldschmidt, Asaf. *The Evolution of Chinese Medicine: Song Dynasty, 960–1200.* London: Roudledge, Taylor & Francis Group, 2009.

Goler, Robert I. "The Marriage of Asclepius and Clio: Recent Studies in the Health Sciences of Early America," *Trends in History*, pp. 55–79.

Grant, Joanna. *A Chinese Physician: Wang Ji and the 'Stone Mountain Medical Case Histories.*' London: Routledge Curzon, 2003.

Greene, Rebecca ed. *History of Medicine. Trends in History*, vol. 4, nos. 2/3. New York: The Institute for Research in History and the Haworth Press, 1988.

Gu, Jiegang 顧頡剛 and Yang Xiangkui 楊向奎. "Sanhuang kao" 三皇考 (A Study of the Three Emperors) In *Gu shi bian* 古史辨 v.7 *zhong*. Lü Simian 呂思勉 and Tong Shuye 童書業 edited. Taibei: Minglun chuban she, 1971.

Gu, Lu 顧祿 comp. *Qingjialu* 清嘉錄. Printed 1830. Lai Xinxia ed. Shanghai: Shanghai guji chubanshe,1986.

Gu, Zhentao 顧震濤. *Wumen biaoyin* 吳門表隱.(Manifesting the Obscure in Suzhou) 1834 edition. Nanjing: Jiangsu guji chubanshe, 1986.

Guangfu zhi 光福志 (Gazetter of the Guangfu region). 1929 edition.

Gusuzhi 姑蘇志 (Gazetter of the Guxu region).

Guo, Aichun 郭靄春, *Zhongguo fensheng yijikao* 中國分省醫籍考 (A Study of Medical Works in China According to Provinces). Vols.1,2. Tianjin: Tianjin kexue jishu chubanshe, 1984 & 1987.

Hang, Shijun 杭世駿. "Yi sanshi shuo" 醫三世說 (A Discourse on the Three Generations in Medicine) in *Daogutang wenji* 道古堂文集 (Collected Essays of the Daogu Studio), 1776 edition.

Hanson, Marta. *Inventing a Tradition in Chinese Medicine: From Universal Canon to Local Medical Knowledge in South China, the Seventeenth to the Nineteenth Century.* PhD Dissertation. University of Pennsylvania, 1997.

——— "Robust Northerners and Delicate Southerners: The Nineteenth-Century Invention of a Southern Medical Tradition." *Positions* 6.3 (Winter 1998): 515–550.

Harper, Donald. *Early Chinese Medical Literature: The Mawangdui Medical Manuscripts.* London: Kegan Paul International, 1998.

Henderson, James. "The Medicine and Medical Practice of the Chinese." *Journal of the North-China Branch of the Royal Asiatic Society*. Vol. 1 (December 1864): 61–105.

Hinrichs, T.J. *The Medical Transforming of Governance and Southern Customs in Song Dynasty China, 960–1279.* PhD Dissertation, Harvard University, 2003.

Ho, Ping-ti. *The Ladder of Success in Imperial China, 1368–1911*. New York: Columbia University Press,1962.

——— *Studies on the Population of China, 1368–1953.*Cambridge: Harvard University Press, 1959.

Hong, Huanchun 洪煥椿. "Lun Ming Qing Suzhou diqu huiguan de xingzhi ji qi zuoyong"論明清蘇州地區會館的性質及其作用 (A Discussion on the Nature and Uses of Local Guilds in Suzhou during the Ming and Qing). *Zhongguoshi yanjiu* 中國史研究 (Study of Chinese History) 1980, no.2:3–15.

——— *Ming Qing Suzhou nongcun jingji zhiliao* 明清蘇州農村經濟質料 (Materials on the Economy of Suzhou Villages in the Ming and Qing). Suzhou: Jiangsu guji chubanshe, 1988.

Hsu, Elisbeth. *The Transmission of Chinese Medicine*. Cambridge: Cambridge University Press, 1999.

Huang, Liu-hung. *Fuhui quanshu* 福惠全書(A Complete Book Concerning Happiness and Benevolence: A Manual for Local Magistrates in the Seventeenth Century China). Translated by Djang Chu. Tuscon: University of Arizona Press,1984.

Huang, Philip C.C. *The Peasant Family and Rural Development in the Yangzi Delta, 1350–1988*. Stanford: Stanford University Press, 1990.

Huang ming jing shi wen bian 皇明經世文編 (Collected Ming Dynasty Writings on Statecraft). Chen, Zilong 陳子龍 compiled. Ming Zhongzheng edition. 30v. Taibei: Guolian tushu chuban, 1964.

Hucker, Charles O. *A Dictionary of Official Titles in Imperial China*. Stanford: Stanford University Press, 1985.

Hymes, Robert. "Not Quite Gentlemen? Doctors in Sung and Yuan," *Chinese Science*, 8 (1987): 9–76.

Ihara, Hiroshi 伊原弘. *Soshû* 蘇州 (Suzhou). Tokyo: Kodansha, 1993.

Imura, Kôzen 井村哮全. Chihôshi ni kisaiseraretaru Chûgoku ekirei ryakkô 地方史に記載せられたる中國疫癘略考 (A Brief Studyof Epidemics in China According to Records of the Local Gazetteers) *Chûgai Iji Shimpô* 中外醫事新報.In eight parts, 1936–37.

Jia, Dedao 賈得道. *Zhongguo yixueshilue* 中國醫學史略(A Short History of Chinese Medicine). Taiyuan: Shanxi renmin chubanshe, 1979.

Jiang, Tingxi 蔣廷錫 (1669–1732) ed. *Gujin tushu jicheng* 古今圖書集成 (Collection of Works Past and Present), 1726 edition. Shanghai: zhonghuashudian, 1934.

Jin, Shoushan , "Woguo zuizao de yixue zazhi: Wuyihuijiang" 我國最早的醫學雜誌: 吳醫匯講 (China's Earliest Medical Journal—the *Wuyi huijiang*).*Zhongyi zazhi* 中醫雜誌 (Chinese Medical Journal). 25.1(1985): 70–71.

Johnson, Linda Cooke ed. *Cities in Jiangnan in Late Imperial China*. New York: State University of NewYork Press, 1993.

Kaptchuk, Ted. *The Web That Has No Weaver: Understanding Chinese Medicine*. New York: Congdon & Weed, 1983.

Ke, Qin 柯琴. *Shanghan laisuji* 傷寒來蘇集 (Renewal of Treatise on Shanghan Illnesses). Preface 1729. Shanghai: Kexue jishu chubanshe, 1986.

Kleinman, Arthur, Peter Kunstadter, E. Russell Alexander, and James L. Gale ed. Medicine in Chinese Cultures: Comparative Studies of Health Care in Chinese and Other Societies. Washington D.C.: Geographic Health Studies, 1975.

Ko, Dorothy. *Teachers of the Inner Chambers: Women and Culture in Seventeenth-Century China*. Stanford: Stanford University Press, 1994.

Kosa, J. "Entrepreneurship and Charisma in the Medical Profession," *Social Science and Medicine*. 4 (1970): 25–40.

Kuhn, Philip A. *Soulstealers: The Chinese Sorcery Scare of 1768*. Cambridge: Harvard University Press,1990.

Kuhn, Thomas S. *The Essential Tension: Selected Studies in Scientific Tradition and Change*. Chicago: University of Chicago Press, 1977.

Kuriyama, Shigehisa. *The Expressiveness of the Body and the Divergence of Greek and Chinese Medicine*. New York: Zone Books, 1999.

——— "The Imagination of Winds and the Development of the Chinese Conception of the Body." Angela Zito and Tani Barlow eds. *Body, Subject and Power in China*. Chicago: University of Chicago Press, 1994: 23–41.

Leavitt, Judith Walzer. "Medicine in Context: A Review Essay of the History of Medicine," *The American Historical Review* 95 (1990): 1471–1484.

Lee, T'ao. "Medical Ethics in Ancient China." *Bulletin of the History of Medicine*. 13 (1943):268–277.

Legge, James. *The Chinese Classics*, With Translations, Critical and Exegetical Notes, Prolegomena and Copious Indexes. 8v. China, n.p., 1939.

Leslie, Charles ed. *Asian Medical Systems*. Berkeley: University of California Press, 1976.

——— and Allan Young ed. *Paths to Asian Medical Knowledge*. Berkeley: University of California Press, 1992.

Leung, Angela. "Medical Learning from the Song to the Ming." *The Song-Yuan-Ming Transition in Chinese History*, ed. by Paul Jakov Smith and Richard von Glahn. Cambridge: Harvard University Press, 2003, pp. 374–398.

——— "Organized Medicine in Ming-Qing China: State and Private Medical Institutions in the Lower Yangzi Region," *Late Imperial China* 8.1(June 1987): 134–166.

Levenson, Joseph. *Modern China and Its Confucian Past: The Problem of Intellectual Continuity*. New York: Anchor Books, 1964.

Li, Bocong 李伯聰. *Bian Que he Bian Que xuepai yanjiu* 扁鵲和扁鵲學派研究(A study of Bian Que and the School of Bian Que) Xi'an: Shaanxi kexue jishu chubanshe, 1990.

Li, Jingwei 李經緯 and Li Zhidong 李志東. *Zhongguo gudai yixue shilue* 中國古代醫學史略 (A Brief History of Ancient Medicine in China). Hebei: Kexue jishu chubanshe, 1990.

Li, Liangsong 李良松 and Guo Hongtao 郭洪濤 ed. *Zhongguo chuantong wenhua yu yixue* 中國傳統文化與醫學(Traditional Chinese Culture and Medicine). Xiamen: Xiamen daxue chubanshe,1990.

Li, T'ao. "Ten Celebrated Physicians and Their Temples" in *Chinese Medical Journal*, 58 (1940): 267-274.

Li, Yun 李雲 et.al. compiled. *Zhongyi renming cidian* 中醫人名辭典 (Dictionary of Names of Chinese Physicians). Beijing: Guoji wenhua chuban gongsi, 1988.

Li, Zhongzi 李中梓. *Yizong bidu* 醫宗必讀 (An Essential Reading on Medicine). Preface 1637. 2v. Beijing: Zhongguo shudian, 1987.

Liang, Zhangju 梁章鉅. *Langji congtan* 浪跡叢談 in *Liangsi biji* 梁氏筆記 (Notes of Mr. Liang), 1918 edition.

Lidai zhongyi zhenben jicheng 歷代中醫珍本集成(Collection of Precious Volumes of Chinese Medicine from Each Dynasty). 40 v. Shanghai:Shanghai sanlian shudian, 1990.

Liu, Guojun 劉國鈞, "Song-Yuan-Ming-Qing di keshu shiye" 宋元明清的刻書事業 (The Profession of Book Printing in Song-Yuan-Ming-Qing) in Zhongguo tushushi ziliaoji 中國圖書史資料集 (Collection of Materials on the History of Books in China) edited by Liu Jiabi 劉家璧. Hong Kong: Longmeng shudian,1974: 481–498.

Liu, Kwang-ching ed. *Orthodoxy in Late Imperial China*, Berkeley: University of California Press, 1990.

Lo, Vivienne. *The Influence of Western Han Nurturing Life Literature on the Development of Acumoxa Therapy*. PhD Dissertation. London University, 1998.

Lu, Maoxiu 陸懋修. *Shibuzhai yishu* 世補齋醫書 (Medical Works from the Shibu Studio). 1884 edition.

——— *Suzhou Chang-Yuan-Wu sanyi kedipu* 蘇州長元吳三邑科第譜 (Genealogy of Graduates ofSecond and Third Degrees from the Three Districts of Changzhou, Yuanhe, and Wu of Suzhou Prefecture). 1906 edition.

Lu, Yitian 陸以湉. *Lenglu yihua* 冷盧醫話 (Medical Discourse from the Lenglu Studio). Preface 1858.

——— Lenglu y*ihua kaozhu* 冷盧醫話考註 (Annotated Medical Discourse from the Lenglu Studio).Annotated by Zhu Weichang 朱偉常. Shanghai: Shanghai Zhongyi xueyuan, 1993.

Marmé Michael. "Population and Possibility in Ming (1368–1644) Suzhou: A Quantified Model," *Ming Studies* 12 (Spring 1981): 29–64.

Mann, Susan. *The Talented Women of the Zhang Family*. Berkeley: University of California Press, 2007.

McKeown, Thomas. *The Role of Medicine*. London: The Nuffield Provincial Hospitals Trust, 1976.

Meng, Wentong 蒙文通 and Miao Fenglin 繆鳳林. "Sanhuang Wudi shuo tan yuan." 三皇五帝說探源 (Seeking the Origins of the Theory on the Three Emperors and Five Rulers) In *Gu shi bian* 古史辨. v.7 *zhong*. Lu Simian 呂思勉 and Tong Shuye 童書業 edited. Taibei: Ming lun chu ban she, 1971.

Miao, Xiyong 繆希雍. *Xianxingzhai yixue guangbiji* 先醒齋醫學廣筆記 (Extensive Notes on Medicine from Xianxing Studio). Printed 1613. Edited based on 1622 edition. Nanjing: Jiangsu kexue jishu chubanshe,1983.

Michihata, Yoshihide 道端良秀. "Tôdai jiin no shaki jigyô: hita yôbyôbô nitsuite" 唐代寺院の社會事業：悲田養病坊に就いて (Social Welfare of the Tang Monasteries-Hospices for the Sick) in *Eizan Gakuhô* 叡山學報 15:18–26.

Minguo Wuxian zhi 民國吳縣志 (Gazetteer of Wu county compiled during the Republican era), 1933 ed. Shanghai: Jiangsu guji chubanshe, 1991.

Ming hui yao 明會要 (MHY)(Collection of Essential Institutions of the Ming). 2v. Shanghai: Zhonghua Shuju, 1957.

Ming shi lu 明實錄 (Veritable Records of the Ming Emperors): *Ming Taizu shilu* 明太祖實錄 (MTZSL); *Ming shizong shilu* 明世宗實錄 (MSZSL); *Ming Muzong shilu* 明穆宗實錄 (MMZSL). Taibei: Institute of History and Philology, Academia Sinica, 1961.

Miyazaki, Ichisada 宮崎市定. *Kakyo* 科舉: Chûgoku no shiken jigoku 中國の試驗地獄 (The Civil Service Examinations: China's Examination Hell) 1963 first edition. Tokyo: Chûô kôronsha, 1986.

——— *Miyazaki Ichisada zenshû* 宮崎市定全集 (The Complete Works of Miyazaki Ichisada). vol.13.Tokyo: Iwanami Shoten, 1992.

Mote, Frederick. "A Millennium of Chinese Urban History: Form, Time, and Space Concepts in Soochow." *Rice University Studies*, 59.4 (1973):35–65.

Naba, Toshisada 那波利貞. "Tôchô seifu no iryô kikô to minshû no jippei ni taisuru kyûsai hôhô ni tsuite no shôkô" 唐朝政府の醫療機構と民衆の疾病に對する救災方法についての小考 (A Brief survey of the Tang Government's Medical Institutions and Measures to Relieve the Populace' Problem of Illness) in *Shisô* 史窗 17.8:1–34.

Naquin, Susan. *Peking: Temples and City Life, 1400-1900.* Berkeley: University of California Press, 2000.

Needham, Joseph. *Clerks and Craftsmen in China and the West*. Cambridge: Cambridge University Press,1970.

Nivinson, David S. and Arthur F. Wright ed. *Confucianism in Action.* Stanford: Stanford University Press, 1959.

Ôba, Osamu 大庭修. Tôsen shinkô kaitôroku 唐船進港回棹錄 (Record of Chinese Ships Coming into Harbor). Suita-shi: Kansai daigaku tozai gakujutsu kenkyûjo, 1974.

Ogawa, Teizo ed. *History of the Professionalization of Medicine. Proceedings of the 3rd International Symposium on the Comparative History of Medicine—East and West.* October 8–14, 1978. Susono-shi, Shizuoka, Japan.

——— ed. *History of Traditional Medicine.Proceedings of the 1st and 2nd International Symposia on the Comparative History of Medicine—East and West*. 1st Symposium: October 22–28,1976. 2nd Symposium: October 23–29, 1977.Susuno-shi, Shizuoka, Japan.

Ôki, Yasushi 大木康, "Minmatsu Kônan ni okeru shuppan bunka no kenkyû 明末江南における出版文化の研究 (A Study of the Print Culture in Late Ming Jiangnan). *Hiroshima daigaku bungakubu kiyô* 廣島大學文學部紀要 50, special issue no. 1(January 1991): 1–176.

Ooms, Herman. *Tokugawa Ideology: Early Constructs,1570–1680*. Princeton: Princeton University Press, 1985.

Ou, Ming 歐明, *Hanying zhongyi cidian* 漢英中醫辭典(Chinese-English Chinese Medical Dictionary). Hong Kong: Sanlian shudian, 1988.

Ouyang, Xiu 歐陽修. *Xintangshu* 新唐書 (The New History of the Tang Dynasty). 20 v. Shanghai: Xinhua shudian, 1975.

Peng, Shaosheng 彭紹升. *Er lin ju ji* 二林居集 2v. Guangxu edition. Taibei: Shimen tushu, 1976.

Peterson, M. Jeanne. *The Medical Profession in Mid-Victorian London*. Berkeley: University of California Press, 1978.

Peterson, Willard J. *The Cambridge History of China*: *The Ch'ing Empire to 1800*. v.9 Part One. Cambridge: Cambridge University Press, 2002.

Pollak, Kurt and E. Ashworth Underwood. *The Healers: The Doctor, Then and Now*. New Jersey: Thomson Nelson and Sons Ltd., 1968.

Porkert, Manfred. *The Theoretical Foundations of Chinese Medicine: Systems of Correspondence*. Cambridge: The MIT Press, 1978.

Porter, Roy. *Doctor of Society*: *Thomas Beddoes and the Sick Trade in Late-Enlightenment England*. NewYork: Routledge, 1992.

——— *Health for Sale*: *Quackery in England 1660–1850*. Manchester: Manchester University Press, 1989.

Porter, Roy ed. *The Popularization of Medicine 1650–1850*. New York: Routledge, 1992.

Qian Gu 錢穀 compiled. *Wu du wen cui xu ji* 吳都文粹續集. n.d. Wenyuange siku quanshu edition. Shanghai: The Commercial Press, 1935.

Qian, Yuanming 錢遠銘 et.al. ed. *Jinshibaijia yilu* 經史百家醫錄 (Medical Collection from the Hundred Schools in the Classics and Histories). Guangzhou: Guangdong keji chubanshe, 1986.

Qiantang xianzhi 錢塘縣志 (Gazetteer of Qiantang county). 1718 preface edition. Tokyo Naikaku Bunko, 1972.

Qingchao tongdian 清朝通典 (Complete Institutions of the Qing Dynasty). Shanghai: The Commercial Press,1935.

Qingchao wenxian tongkao 清朝文獻通考 (Complete Examination of Qing Dynasty Documents).Shanghai: Shangwuin shuguan, 1936.

Qingshigao 清史稿 (Draft of Qing Dynasty history). Beijing: Zhonghua shuju, 1976–77.

Rankin, Mary. *Elite Activitism and Political Transformation in China, Zhejiang Province, 1865–1911*. Stanford: Stanford University Press, 1986.

Ren, Xigeng 任錫庚. "Taiyiyuan zhi" 太醫院志 (An Annal of the Imperial Medical Academy," in *Qingdai zhanggu zhuilu* 清代掌故綴錄 (A Collection of Historical Records of the Qing Dynasty). Edited by Zhou Kangxie 周康燮. Chongwen shudian, 1971.

Ren, Yingqiu 任應秋. *Zhongyi gejia xueshuo* 中醫各家學說(Theories of Different Schools in Traditional Chinese Medicine). Shanghai: Kexue jishu chubanshe, 1980.

Risse, Guenter. *Hospital Life in Enlightenment Scotland*. Cambridge: Cambridge University Press,1986.

Rosenberg, Charles. *The Care of Strangers: The Rise of America's Hospital System*. New York: Basic Books,1987.

——— "Disease in History: Frames and Framers," *Milbank Quarterly*, 67, supplement 1 (1989): 1–15.

——— *Explaining Epidemics and Other Studies in the History of Medicine*. Cambridge: Cambridge University Press, 1992.

Rowe, William T. *Hankow: Commerce and Society in a Chinese City, 1796–1889*. Stanford: Stanford University Press, 1984.

——— *Hankow: Conflict and Community in a Chinese City, 1796–1895*. Stanford: Stanford University Press, 1989.

Rugoff, Milton ed. *The Travels of Marco Polo*. New York: New American Library, 1986.

Rumen shiqin jiaozhu 儒門事親校註 (Annotated Commentary of Confucian's Duties to Their Parents). 1228. By Zhang, Congzheng 張從正. Zhengzhou: Henan kexue jishu chubanshe, 1984.

Scheid, Volker. *Currents of Tradition in Chinese Medicine, 1626–2006*. Seattle: Eastland Press, 2007.

Shen, Shiyu 沈時譽. *Yiheng* 醫衡 (Physician as the Authority). Published 1661. Shanghai: Xinghua shudian, 1985.

Shen, Xieyuan 沈燮元. "Mingdai Jiangsu keshu shiye gaishu"明代江蘇刻書事業概述 (A Brief Account of the Profession of Book Publishing in Jiangsu during the Ming). *Lidai keshu gaikuang* 歷代刻書概況.Beijing: Yinshua gongye chubanshe, 1991: 309–317.

Shi, Shoutang 石壽棠. *Yiyuan* 醫原 (Origins of Medicine). Printed 1861. Nanjing: Jiangsu guji chubanshe, 1983.

Shinno, Reiko. "Medical Schools and the Temples of the Three Progenitors in Yuan China: A Case of Cross-Cultural Interactions." *Harvard Journal of Asiatic Studies* volume 67. 1 (June 2007): 89–133

Sigerist, Henry E. "The Social History of Medicine," *Henry E. Sigerist on the History of Medicine*, Felix Marti-Ibanez ed. New York: M.D. Publications, 1960: 25–33.

Sima, Qian 司馬遷. *Shiji* 史記 (Historical Records).10v. Beijing: Zhonghua shuju, 1975.

Siku quanshu zongmu tiyao 四庫全書總目提要 (An Abstract of the Index to the Complete Works of The Four Divisions) 4 v. Shanghai: The Commercial Press, 1933.

Sima, Qian 司馬遷. *Shiji* 史记 (Records of History). 10v. Beijing: Zhonghua shuju, 1975

Siraisi, Nancy. *Medieval and Early Renaissance Medicine: An Introduction to Knowledge and Practice*. Chicago: University of Chicago Press,1990.

Sishu jizhu 四書集註 (Collected Annotation of the Four Books). Zhu Xi 朱熹. Taibei: Shijie shuju, 1985.

Sivin, Nathan. "Ailment and Cure in Traditional China: An Anthropological Study of Classical and Popular Medicine before Modern Times, with Implications for the Present." Unpublished Manuscript.

——— "Science and Medicine in Chinese History," *Heritage of China: Contemporary Perspectives on Chinese Civilization*. Paul S. Ropp ed. Berkeley: University of California Press, 1990: 164–196.

——— "Science and Medicine in Imperial China—The State of the Field," *The Journal of Asian Studies*, 47.1 (February 1988): 41–90.

——— "Social Relations of Curing in Traditional China: Preliminary Considerations," *Nihon ishigaku zasshi* 日本醫史學雜誌 (Journal of the Japan Society of Medical History)23.4 (October 1977): 1–28.

——— *Traditional Medicine in Contemporary China*. Ann Arbor: The University of Michigan Press,1987.

Song, Lian 宋濂. *Song Wenxiangong Quanji* 宋文憲公全集, juan 44 in *SibuBeiyao*.

Smith, Hilary. *Foot Qi: History of A Chinese Medical Disorder*. PhD Dissertation. University of Pennsylvania, 2008.

Smith, Richard. "Ritual in Ch'ing Culture." In *Orthodoxy in Late Imperial China*. Ed. by Kwang-ching Liu. Berkeley: University of California Press, 1990.

Spence, Jonathan D. *Emperor of China, Self Portrait of K'ang-hsi*. New York: Vintage Books, 1988.

Spink, Wesley W. *Infectious Diseases: Prevention and Treatment in the Nineteenth and Twentieth Centuries*. Minneapolis: University of Minnesota Press, 1978.

Stevenson, Lloyd G. "A Second Opinion," *Bulletin of the History of Medicine*, 54 (1980): 134–40.

Su, Tiege 蘇鐵戈. "Wuyi Huijiang wei lianxu chuban kanwu zhi zhiyi" 吳醫匯講為連續出版刊物之質疑 (On the Question of Wuyi Huijiang as a Consecutive Publication). *Zhonghua yishi zazhi* 中華醫史雜誌(Chinese Medical Journal) 1993, 23.3:145–148.

Sun, Chengze 孫承澤. *Chun ming meng yu lu.* 春明夢餘錄. Based on Qianlong edition. Beijing: Guji Chubanshe, 1992.

Sun, Zigao 孫子高 "Sanhuang kao 三皇考" (A Study of the Three Emperors) In *Tushu jikan* 圖書季刊. V. 3 no.12 (March 1936): 783-787.

Suzhou fu zhi 蘇州府志 (Gazetteer of Suzhou). 6v. Taibei: Chenwen chubanshe, 1970.

Suzhou zhizao Li Xu zouzhe 蘇州織造李煦奏摺 (Memorials of the Suzhou Superintendent of Imperial Silk Manufacturing Li Xu). Taibei: Wenhai chubanshe,1977.

Tamba no Mototane 丹波元胤 compiled. *Zhongguo yijikao* 中國醫籍考 (A Study of Chinese Medical Texts).Published 1826. Beijing: Renmin weisheng chubanshe, 1983.

Tang, Dalie 唐大烈 comp. *Wuyi huijiang* 吳醫匯講(Collected discourses of Suzhou physicians) Ding Guangdi ed. based on 1814 edition, with reference to 1792 and later editions. Shanghai: Xinhua shudian, 1983.

Taylor, Kim. *Chinese Medicine in Early Communist China,1945–1963: Medicine of Revolution.* London: Routledge Curzon, 2004.

Tsu, Yu-yue. *The Spirit of Chinese Philanthropy: A Study in Mutual Aid.* London: Longmans, Green &Co., Agents, 1912.

Twitchett, Dennis and John K. Fairbank ed. *The Cambridge History of China*, v.9, Part One: *The Ch'ing Empire to 1800*. Cambridge: Cambridge University Press, 2002.

Unschuld, Paul U. Translated and Annotated. *Forgotten Traditions of Ancient Chinese Medicine: The I-hsüeh yüan liu lun of 1757 by Hsü Ta-ch'un.* Massachusetts: Paradigm Publications, 1990.

——— *Huang Di nei jing su wen: Nature: Knowledge, Imagery in an Ancient Chinese Medical Text* . Berkeley: University of California Press, 2003.

——— *Medical Ethics in Imperial China: A Study in Historical Anthropology*. Berkeley: University of California Press, 1979.

———. *Medicine in China: A History of Pharmaceutics*. Berkeley: University of California Press, 1986.

——— "Traditional Chinese Medicine: Some Historical and Epistemological Reflections," *Social Science and Medicine*, 24.12 (1987): 1023–1029.

Von Glahn, Richard. *Fountain of Fortune: Money and Monetary Policy in China,1000–1700.* Berkeley: University of California Press, 1996.

——— *The Sinister Way: The Divine and the Demonic in Chinese Religious Culture.* Berkeley: University of California Press, 2004.

Vollmer, Howard M. and Donald L. Mills, eds. *Professionalization*. Englewood Cliffs, 1966.

Wang Ao 王鏊 comp. *Gusu zhi* 姑蘇志 (Gazetteer of the Gusu region). Wenyuange edition. Siqu quanshu chenben shiji, Taibei: The Commercial Press, 1980.

Wang, Dexuan 王德宣. *Wenbing zhengzong* 溫病正宗 (The Orthodox Teachings of *Wenbing*). Edited based on 1936 edition. Beijing: Zhongyi guji chubanshe, 1987.

Wang, Kentang 王肯堂. *Wang Kentang jianshi* 王肯堂箋釋(Commentary Explanations by Wang Kentang). 1689 edition.

Wang, Lun 王綸. *Mingyi zazhu* 明醫雜著 (Collection of Miscellaneous Experiences of Ming Physicians).1551 edition. Nanjing: Jiangsu kexue jishu chubanshe, 1985.

Wang, Pu 王溥 compiled. *Tanghuiyao.* 唐會要 3v. Beijing: Zhonghua shuju, 1955.

Wang, Qi 王圻 compiled. *Xu wenxian tongkao.* 續文獻通考 (Comprehensive Study of Documents, Supplements) Wanli edition. 24v. Taibei: Wenhai chuban she, 1981.

Wang, Wei 王褘. "Lun yi" 論醫 (Discourse on Physicians). GJTSJC Yibu quanlu 古今圖書集成醫部全錄 (Collection of Works Past and Present: Complete Collection of the Medical Section) 518:434.

Wang, Zijie 王子接. *Jiangxueyuan gufang xuanzhu* 絳雪園古方選注 (Selected Annotation on Ancien Formulae from the Jiangxue Garden). Published1732. Edited by Li Fei 李飛 based on the 1737edition. Shanghai: Shanghai Kexue jishu chubanshe, 1982.

Wei Yinru 魏隱儒, *Zhongguo shuji yinshuashi* 中國書籍印刷史 (The History of Book Printing inChina). Beijing: Yinshua gongye chubanshe, 1984.

Wenyilun pingzhu 溫疫論評注 (Commentary on the Treatise on Warm Factor Epidemic Disorders). 2nd printing. Beijing: Renmin weisheng chubanshe, 1985.

Will, Pierre-Etienne. *Bureaucracy* and Famine in Eighteenth-Century China. Translated from the French by Elborg Forster. Stanford: Stanford University Press, 1990.

Will, Pierre-Etienne and R. Bin Wong. *Nourish the People: The State Civilian Granary System in China, 1650–1850.* Michigan: Center for Chinese Studies, The University of Michigan, 1991.

Wilson, Leonard. "Medical History Without Medicine," *Journal of the History of Medicine*, 35 (1980):5–7.

Wilson, Thomas A. *Genealogy of the Way: The Construction and Uses of the Confucian Tradition in Late Imperial China.* Stanford: Stanford University Press, 1995.

——— "The Ritual Formation of Confucian Orthodoxy and the Descendants of the Sage." In *Journal of Asian Studies* 55.3 (August 1996): 559-584.

Wong, K. Chimin and Wu Lien-teh. *History of Chinese Medicine: Being a Chronicle of Medical Happenings in China from Ancient Times to the Present Period.* Shanhgai: National Quarantine Service, 1936.

Wu, Ceng 吳曾. *Nenggai zhai manlu* 能改齋漫錄 (Leisure Notes from the Nenggai Studio). *Mohai jinhu* 墨海金壺 (Golden Vase in the Sea of Ink) (Shanghai: Bogu zhai, 1921). Vols. 80–83.

Wu, Cheng 吳澄. *Wu Wenzheng ji* 吳文正集(Collected Writings of Wu Wenzheng). *Ying yin Wen yuan ge Si ku quan shu*, v.1197. Taibei: The Commercial Press, 1983.

Wu, Kaopan 吳考槃. "Huangdi Neijing, Suwen, Lingshu kao" 《黃帝內經》《素問》《靈樞》考 (A Study of the Canon of the Yellow Emperor, Suwen and Lingshu). *Zhonghua yishi zazhi*. 13.2 (1983): 85–87.

Wu, Yili. "The Bamboo Grove Mnastery and Popular Gynecology in Qing China." *Late Imperial China* 21.1 (June 2000): 41–76.

——— *Transmitted Secrets: The Doctors of the Lower Yangzi Region and Popular Gynecology in Late Imperial China.* PhD Dissertation. Yale University. 1998.

Wu, Youxing 吳有性. *Wenyilun* 瘟疫論 (Treatise on Warm Factor Epidemic Disorders). Preface 1642. Hong Tianci commentary. 1842 edition.

Wuxian zhi 吳縣志 (Gazetteer of Wu county). 1691edition. Yangzhou: Guangling guji, 1989.

Xiao, Jing 蕭京. *Xuanqi jiuzhenglun* 軒歧救正論 (Discourse on Rectification According to the Yellow Emperor's Treatise) Preface 1644. Beijing: Zhongyi guji chubanshe, 1983.

Xie, Guan 謝觀. Zhongguo yixue dacidian 中國醫學大辭典(Cyclopedia of Chinese Medicine). 2v. 5thedition. Shanghai: The Commercial Press, 1927.

Xingan huilan 刑案匯覽 (Conspectus of Penal Cases).1886 edition. Taibei: Chengwen chubanshe, 1967.

Xu, Dachun 徐大椿. *Huixi yian* 洄溪醫案 (Medical Cases of Huixi). Preface 1855. *Yixue Yuanliu lun* 醫學源流論 (Discourse on the Source and History of Medicine). Author preface 1757. Beijing: Zhongguo shudian, 1987.

——— *Shenji Chuyan* 慎疾芻言 (Plain Talk on Caution on Illnesses). Preface 1767. *Yijing shuohuijiji qita erzhong* 醫經溯洄集及其他二種 (Collection on Tracing the Sources of the Medical Classics and Two Other Kinds). Shanghai: The Commercial Press,1937.

Xu, Dixin 許滌新 and Wu Chengming 吳承明. *Zhongguo zibenchuyi di mengya* 中國資本主義的萌芽 (The Sprouts of Capitalism in China). Beijing: Renmin chubanshe, 1985.

Yamada, Keiji 山田慶兒. "The Formation of the *Huang-ti Nei-ching*." *Acta Asiatica* 36 (1979): 67-89.

——— *Yorunaku Tori* 夜鳴く鳥.Tokyo: Iwanami shoten, 1990.

Yamamoto, Noriko 山本徳子. "Chûgoku no Kotowaza wo tsujiteno ishazô," 中国の諺を通じての医者像 (Portrait of Physicians as seen from the Chinese Proverbs) *Nihon ishigaku zasshi* 日本醫史學雜誌 (Journal of the Japan Society of Medical History). 23.2 (April1977): 172–174.

Yan, Shiyi 嚴世藝. *Zhongyi xueshushi* 中醫學術史 (A History of the Scholarship of Traditional Chinese Medicine) Shanghai: Zhongyi xueyuan chubanshe,1989.

Yang, Jialuo 楊家駱. *Shitong fenlei zongzuan* 十通分類總纂(Combined Collection of the Classified Ten Encyclopaedic Histories of Institutions). Taibei: Dingwen shuju, 1975.

Yazawa, Toshihiko 矢沢利彦 translated. Chûgoku no yigaku to gijitsu: Iyezusu kaishi shokanshu 中國の醫学と技術: イエズス會士書簡集. Lettres edifiantes et curieuses, ecrites des Missions Etrangeres. (Letters of the Jesuit Missions, Medicine and Technology of China) Nouvelle edition. 26 vols. Paris 1780–1783. Sections on Medicine. Tokyo: Tôyô bunko, 1977.

Ye, Dehui 葉德輝. *Shulin qinghua* 書林清話 (Pure Talk on Bookstores). 1910 edition.

Ye, Tianshi 葉天士. *Linzheng zhinan yian* 臨証指南醫案(Case Reports for Guide to Clinical Practice).1764. Commentary by Xu Lingtai 徐靈胎. Shanghai:Renmin chubanshe, 1976.

Ye, Yiting 葉怡庭 edited. *Lidai yixue mingzhu xuji pingshi* 歷代醫學名著序集評史 (Comments and Explanations on the Prefaces of Famous Medical Classics throughout the Dynasties). Shanghai: Kexue jixshu chubanshe, 1987.

Yi jian zhi 夷堅志. 1879 preface. 十萬卷樓叢書 edition.叢書集成. Shanghai: Shangwuin shuguan, 1937.

Yongzhen zghupi yuzhi 雍正硃批諭旨 (Vermillion Edicts of the Yongzheng Emperor).

You, Cheng 尤乘. *Shoushi qingpian* 壽世青篇 (An Essay on Longevity), 1667. *Zhenben yishu jicheng* 14.Shanghai: Shanghai kexue jishu chubanshe, 1986.

You, Yi 尤怡. *Shanghan guanzhuji* 傷寒貫珠集(Collection of Precious Materials on Cold Damaged Disorders). 1810. 3rd printing. Shanghai:Shanghai kexue jishu chubanshe, 1978.

——— *Yixue dushu ji* 醫學讀書記 (Record of Studying Medicine) Based on 1814 edition and edited with 1884 and 1936 editions. Beijing: Renmin weishen chubanshe, 1991.

Yu, Chang 喻昌. *Shanglun pian* 尙論篇 (An Essay on Respectful Discourse). Printed 1648. *Sikuquanshu zhenben erji* 四庫全書珍本二集. Vols. 192–193.

——— *Yimen Falü* 醫門法律 (The Laws of Medicine).*Sikuquanshu Zhenben Erji* 四庫全書珍本二集. Vols.194–195.

Yu, Ji 虞集. *Dao yuan xue gu lu* 道園學古錄. Ming edition. Sibu Congkan. Shanghai: The Commercial Press, 1967.

Yü, Yingshi 余英時. *Zhongguo sixiang chuantong de xiandai quanshi* 中國思想傳統的現代詮釋 (A Contemporary Interpretation of Chinese Intellectual Tradition). Taibei: Lianking chubanshe, 5th printing, 1992.

Yuan Mei 袁枚. *Xiaocangshanfang wenji* 小倉山房文集(Collected Prose from the Hut on Mount Xiaocang) *Suiyuan quanji* 隋園全集 (Complete Collection of the Sui Gardens). 1918 edition.

Yuan, Shouding 袁守定. *Tumin lu* 圖民錄. 1872 edition.

Yuanhe xianzhi 元和縣志 (Gazetteer of Yuanhe county).1761 edition. Yangzhou: Guangling guji, 1989.

Yuan shi 元史 (History of Yuan). Song, Lian 宋濂 compiled. Beijing: Zhonghua Shuju,

Zha, Jizuo 查繼佐. *Zuiweilu* 罪惟錄 (Record of Solemn Sins). 4v. Zhejiang: Zhejiang guji chubanshe, 1986

Zhang, Cai 張采. *Zhiweitang wencun* 知畏堂文存(Preserved Essays from the Zhiwei Hall). Preface dated 1674. 1965 Library of Congress photocopy of the National Beijing Library edition.

Zhang, Jiebin 張介賓. *Jingyue quanshu* 景岳全書 (The Complete Works of Jingyue). 1711 edition. Shanghai: Shanghai kexue jixhu chubanshe, 1959.

Zhang, Lu 張璐. *Zhangshi Yitong* 張氏醫通 (Zhang's Treatise on General Medicine) 1719 preface edition, Shanghai: Shanghai kexue jishu chubanshe, 1963.

Zhang, Tingyu 張廷玉. *Ming shi* 明史 (History of Ming).28 v. Beijing: Zhonghua shuju, 1974.

Zhang, Zhicong 張志聰 and Gao Shishi 高士栻. *Lüshan yichao* 侶山醫鈔 (Medical Notes from L han). Original Preface by Zhang Zhicong dated 1699.Taibei: Tianyi chubanshe, 1973.

Zhang, Zhihan 張知寒 and Du Guanhua 杜冠華. "Yiru guanxi luelun" 醫儒關係略論 (A Brief Discourse on the Relationship between Confucianism and Medicine). *Zhonghua yishi zazhi* 中華醫史雜誌.23.2 (1993): 69–71.

Zhang, Xuecheng 章學誠. *Bingchen zhaji* 丙辰劄記. In Zhang Shizhai zha ji si zhong 章實齋扎記 四種. Taibei: Guangwen shuju, 1971.

Zhang Zhongjing 張仲景. *Shanghan lun* 傷寒論 (Treatise on Febrile Diseases Caused by Cold.). Translated by Luo Xiwen. Beijing: New World Press, 1986.

Zhao, Xuemin 趙學敏. *Chuanya neipian* 串雅內篇 (The Inner Essay of the Principle Book of Quackery). 1890 edition.

Zhenben yishu jicheng 珍本醫書集成 (Collection of Precious Works on Medicine). Shanghai: Shanghai kexue jishu chubanshe, 1985.

Zheng, Jinsheng 鄭金生. "Zhongguo lidai yaowang ji yaowang miao tanyuan" 中國歷代藥王及藥王廟探源 (Probing the Origin of Chinese Medical Kings and Temples of Medical Kings of Successive Ages) in *Zhonghua yishi zazhi* 中華醫史雜誌, 26:2 (April, 1996): 65–72.

Zhongguo wenhua jinghua quanji: yixue juan 中國文化精華全集：醫學卷 (Complete Collection ofthe Essence of Chinese Culture: Medicine).Beijing: Zhongguo guoji guangbo chubanshe, 1992.

Zhu, Yizun 朱彝尊. *Pu shu ting ji* 曝書亭集 (Collected Works from the Pavillion for Drying Books). Siku quanshu edition. Taibei: The Commercial Press, 1983.

Zhu, Zhenheng 朱震亨. *Gezhi yulun* 格致餘論(Supplementary Discussions for the Perfection ofUnderstanding Through the Investigation of Phenomena). 1347. Nanjing: Jiangsu kexue jishu chubanshe, 1985.

INDEX

T

W

Asian Thought and Culture

This series is designed to cover three inter-related projects:

- *Asian Classics Translation*, including those modern Asian works that have been generally accepted as "classics"
- *Asian and Comparative Philosophy and Religion*, including excellent and publishable Ph.D. dissertations, scholarly monographs, or collected essays
- *Asian Thought and Culture in a Broader Perspective*, covering exciting and publishable works in Asian culture, history, political and social thought, education, literature, music, fine arts, performing arts, martial arts, medicine, etc.

For additional information about this series or for the submission of manuscripts, please contact:

Peter Lang Publishing, Inc.
Acquisitions Department
29 Broadway, 18th floor
New York, New York 10006

To order other books in this series, please contact our Customer Service Department at:

800-770-LANG (within the U.S.)
(212) 647-7706 (outside the U.S.)
(212) 647-7707 FAX

Or browse online by series at:

www.peterlang.com